DIAGNOSTIC
Picture Tests
in Clinical Medicine

4 D0685522

G S J Chessell, Dip Ed Tech.
Coordinator, Medical Learning Resources Group,
University of Aberdeen

M J Jamieson, MRCP
Lecturer, Department of Therapeutics and Clinical
Pharmacology, University of Aberdeen

R A Morton, MSc
Director, Department of Medical Illustration,
University of Aberdeen

J C Petrie, FRCP
Reader, Department of Therapeutics and Clinical
Pharmacology, University of Aberdeen; Honorary
Consultant Physician, Aberdeen Teaching
Hospitals.

H M A Towler, MRCP
Lecturer, Department of Medicine,
University of Aberdeen.

NM Mosby-Wolfe

PREFACE

This is volume four of a four-volume series. The aim is to test diagnostic skills over a wide range of clinical problems. Questions which may feature in examinations or in clinical practice are posed in an attempt to stimulate the undergraduate or postgraduate to undertake further reading.

The pictures in this new series have been selected from the clinical slide library in the Department of Medical Illustration, University of Aberdeen. The books have been produced against a background of experience gained over the last 10 years in the compilation for local use of over 2,000 self-assessment examples. The local exercise was coordinated through the Medical Learning Resources Group of the Faculty of Medicine, University of Aberdeen, in collaboration with many of the clinicians in the Aberdeen Teaching Hospitals.

We hope that the books will be of interest to all who are committed to their own continuing medical education. We would welcome comment on individual questions and answers.

GSJC, MJJ, RAM, JCP, HMAT.

Although numbering is sequential, each volume in the series is unique, containing a balanced selection of diagnostic examples, and thus may be used independently.

ACKNOWLEDGEMENTS

We wish to acknowledge the invaluable contribution of Dr Anthony Hedley, now Professor of Community Medicine, University of Glasgow, who was the instigator of the self-assessment programme on which these books are based. We would also like to acknowledge the cooperation of all patients, secretarial and technical staff, in particular the staff of the Department of Medical Illustration, who have contributed in one way or another to the preparation of these volumes, and Mrs Margaret Doverty who typed the manuscript.

We would particularly like to thank the following colleagues for contributing material for the books:

Dr D R Abramovich, Mr A Adam, Mr A K Ah-See, Dr D J G Bain, Dr L S Bain, Dr K Bartlett, Dr A P Bayliss, Dr B Bennett, Miss F M Bennett, Dr P Best, Dr P D Bewsher, Mr C Birchall, Mr C T Blaiklock, Dr L J Borthwick, Mr P L Brunnen, Dr P W Brunt, Dr J Calder, Professor A G M Campbell, Dr B Carrie, Dr P Carter, Dr G R D Catto, Mr R B Chesney, Dr N Clark, Mr P B Clarke, Mr A I Davidson, Dr R J L Davidson, Dr A A Dawson, Mr W B M Donaldson, Professor A S Douglas, Dr A W Downie, Dr C J Eastmond, Mr J Engeset, Dr N Edward, Dr J K Finlayson, Dr J R S Finnie, Mr A V Foote, Dr N G Fraser, Mr R J A Fraser, Dr J A R Friend, Dr D B Galloway, Mr J M C Gibson, Dr D Hadley, Dr J E C Hern, Dr A W Hutcheon, Dr T A Jeffers, Dr A W Johnston, Mr P F Jones, Dr A C F Kenmure, Mr I R Kernohan, Dr A S M Khir, Mr J Kyle, Dr J S Legge, Mr McFadzean, Dr E McKay, Mr J McLauchlan, Mr K A McLay, Professor M MacLeod, Dr R A Main, Mr Mather, Mr N A Matheson, Mr J D B Miller, Mr S S Miller, Mr K L G Mills, Dr N A G Mowat, Mr I F K Muir, Dr L E Murchison, Mr W J Newlands, Mr J G Page, Professor R Postlethwaite, Dr J M Rawles, Mr P K Ray, Mr C R W Rayner, Professor A M Rennie, Mr A G R Rennie, Dr J A N Rennie, Dr O J Robb, Dr H S Ross, Dr G Russell, Dr D S Short, Dr P J Smail, Dr C C Smith, Professor G Smith, Dr L Stankler, Mr J H Steyn, Professor J M Stowers, Dr G H Swapp, Mr J Wallace, Professor W Walker, Dr S J Watt, Dr J Weir, Dr J Webster, Dr M I White, Dr F W Wigzell, Dr M J Williams, Mr L C Wills, Dr L A Wilson, Mr H A Young.

583 These are oriental sores.
  a Which organism is responsible?
  b What is the vector?
  c Is the patient likely to have splenomegaly?
  d Does spontaneous cure occur?

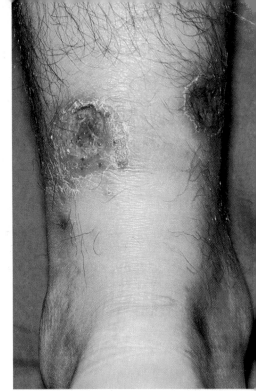

583

584 Name three conditions which may give rise to this appearance.

584

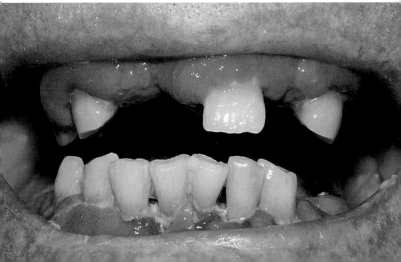

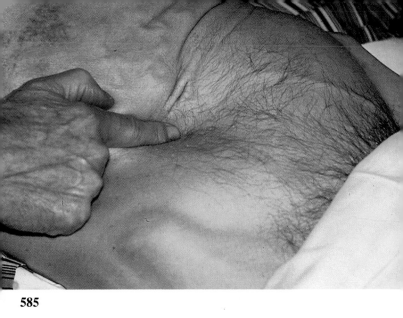

585

585 and 586
    a What principal abnormality is present on this patient's abdomen?
        What feature of this is being demonstrated?
    b What is the likely diagnosis?

586

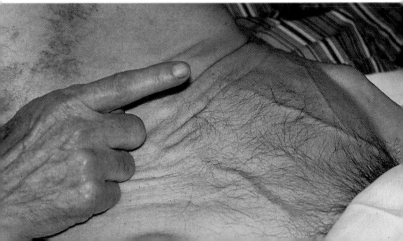

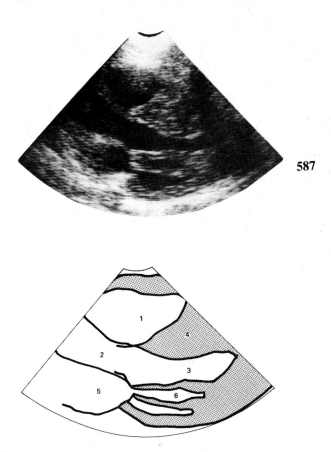

587

587
This long axis cross-sectional echocardiogram is of a twenty-five year old asymptomatic policeman. An abnormal electrocardiogram and a systolic murmur were noted at a routine medical examination.
a Name the structures 1-6 and indicate which of these is abnormal.
b What is the diagnosis?

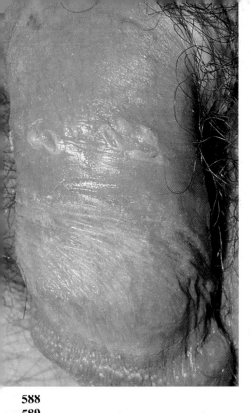

588 a What is the likely causative organism of this painful lesion?
b Why might the patient complain of headache?

589 This patient with psoriasis has recently had surgery.
a What name is given to this appearance?
b In what other conditions may this occur?

588
589

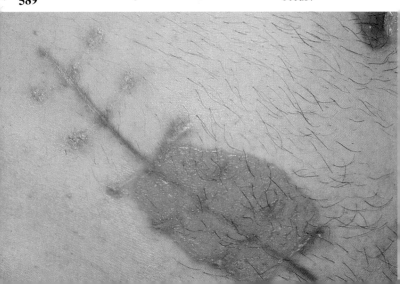

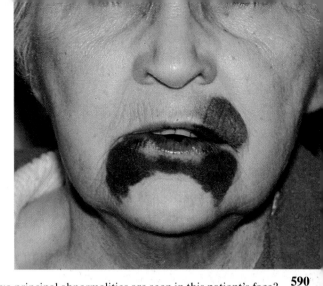

590 a What two principal abnormalities are seen in this patient's face?
b In what two ways may they be related?

591 This patient developed a pruritic eruption over his shoulders, elbows, and knees.
a Why should he have dietary advice?
b Which antibody may be detected in such skin lesions?

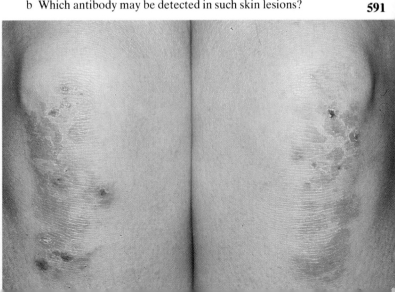

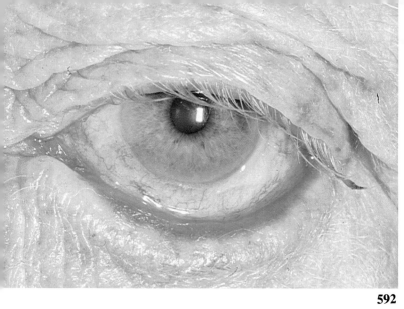

592

592 This patient complains of excessive watering of this eye.
    a What is this condition?
    b What is the usual cause?

593 a What is the diagnosis?
    b What abnormalities might be found in
       i)   the arterial blood pressure?
      ii)   the jugular venous pulse?

593

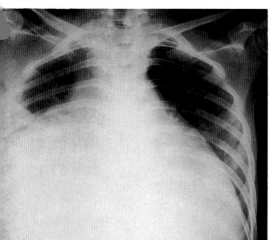

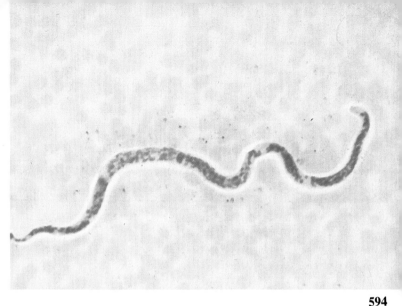

594

594 a What type of organism is seen on this blood film?
   b Name two diseases in which this phase of the organism's life cycle will allow their identification.
   c What abnormality is likely to be found in the differential white cell count?

595 a What radiological abnormality is visible?
   b What is the likely cause?

595

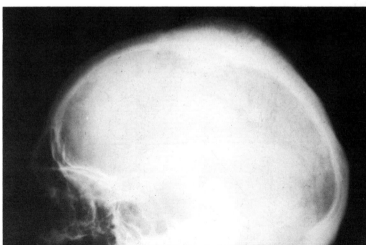

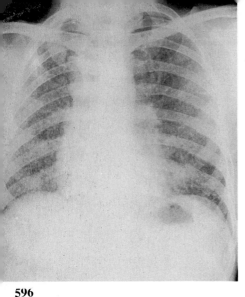

596 This patient gives a two year history of increasing exertional dyspnoea.
  a What abnormality is seen in the lung fields?
  b What abnormalities are likely in pulmonary function tests?

596

597

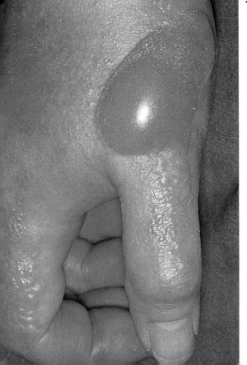

597 This patient was found unconscious.
What cause of her coma is suggested by these appearances?

598 This patient complains of persistent discharge.
   a What is this condition called?
   b What hormonal abnormality is likely?
   c List three drugs that may cause this condition

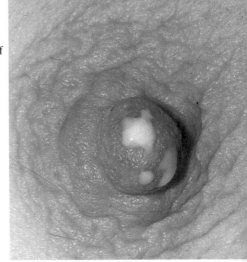

598

599

599 This condition has progressed over three weeks.
   a What is the diagnosis?
   b What is the causative agent?
   c What is likely to be the patient's occupation?

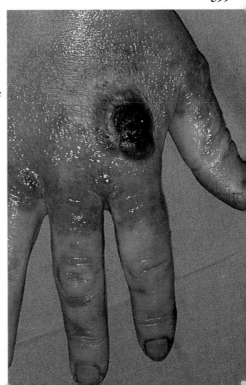

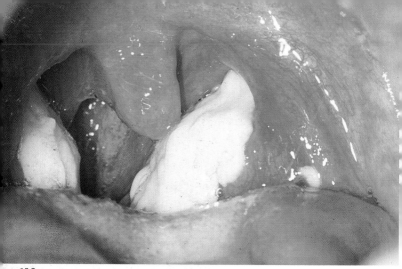

600

601

600 a State two likely causes
for this appearance of
the throat.
b Suggest four
investigations which
may be useful in
establishing these
diagnoses.

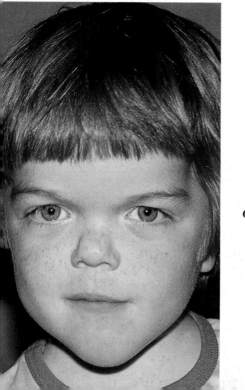

601 This child's height is
consistently below the
third centile for his age.
He was delivered by
Caesarean section.
a What is the diagnosis?
b What is the usual mode
of inheritance of this
condition?
c What is the significance
of the obstetric history?

602 a What facial
abnormalities are
shown?
b What is the likely
diagnosis?
c What single test would
be useful to diagnose
the underlying
aetiology?

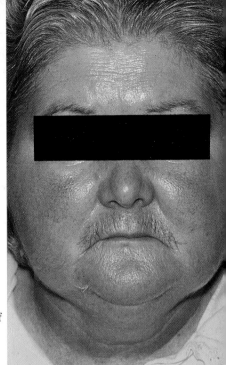

603 This diabetic patient
complains of rapidly
worsening pain and loss of
visual acuity in this eye.
a List three
abnormalities seen
here.
b What is the cause of his
symptoms?

602
603

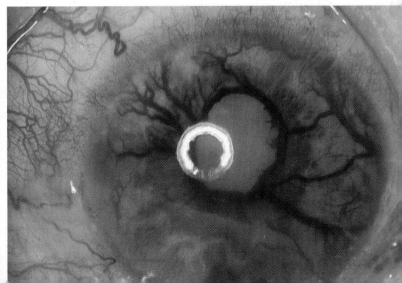

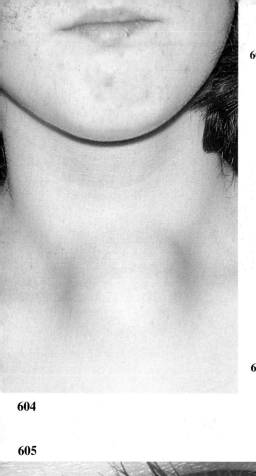

604 a Which two principal alternatives would you consider as causes of this girl's neck swelling?
b How would you distinguish these clinically?

604

605 a What is this?
b With which infectious disease is this characteristically associated?
c What is the causative agent?

605

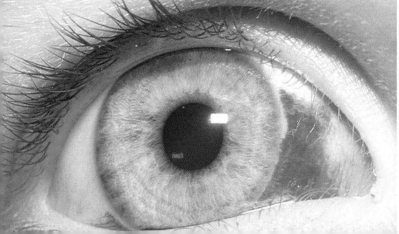

606
This patient experienced
pain behind this eye, with
impaired visual acuity, six
months ago.
a What abnormality is
   shown?
b What condition
   explains his earlier
   symptoms?

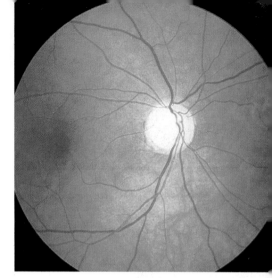

606

607 This girl has secondary
amenorrhoea.
a What abnormality is
   shown?
b Which primarily non-
   endocrine disorder
   does this suggest?

607

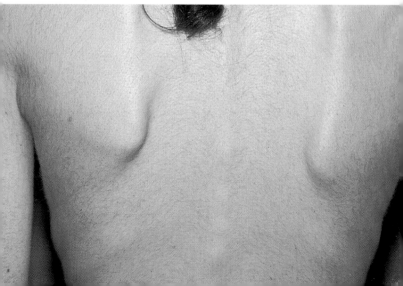

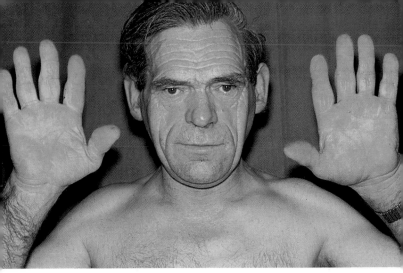

608

609

608 a What is the diagnosis?
b What hormonal abnormalities may this patient have?

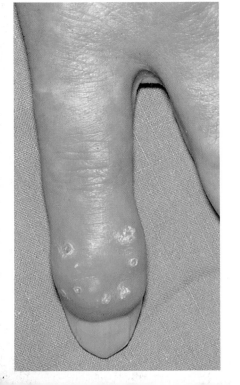

609 a What is this?
b What is the underlying biochemical disorder?
c What are the indications for specific long-term treatment of this disorder?

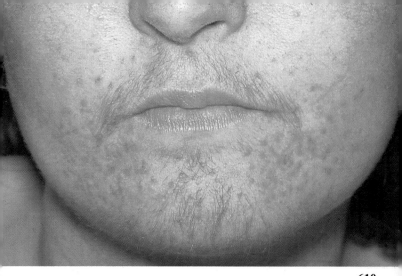

10 a What abnormalities are seen in this female patient's face?
   b List three important causes (of this condition).

610

611

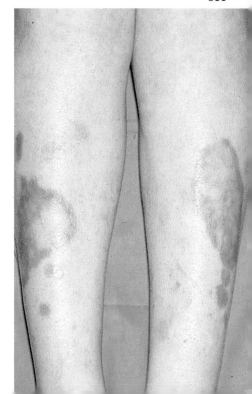

11 This patient presents with a three month history of weight loss and polyuria.
   a What is the skin condition on the patient's shins?
   b What is the underlying diagnosis?

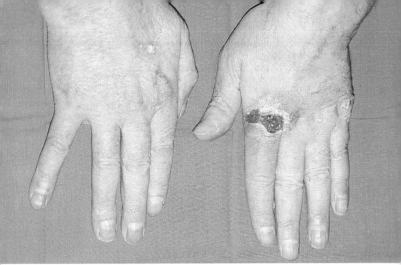

612

612 This patient was in contact with arsenicals during his childhood. What complications have developed?

613

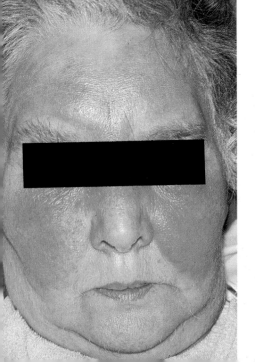

613 a What is the causative organism?
b Is the condition painful?

614 What is the aetiology of this iatrogenic lesion?

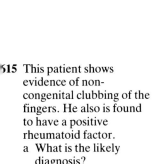

614

615 This patient shows evidence of non-congenital clubbing of the fingers. He also is found to have a positive rheumatoid factor.
a What is the likely diagnosis?
b Does this condition reduce the risk of bronchial carcinoma?

615

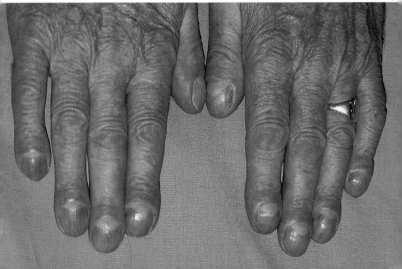

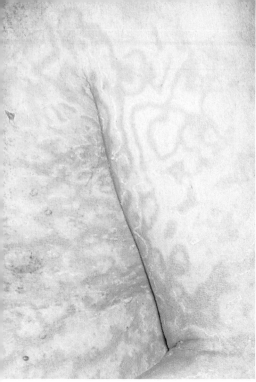

616
This patient's rash is noted to spread, as if in waves, across his body.
a What name is given to this eruption?
b What is its significance?

616

617

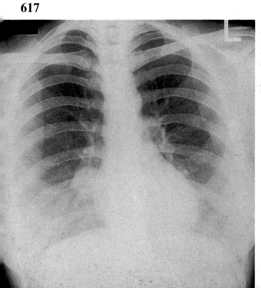

617
This patient has no respiratory symptoms.
a What abnormality is seen in the chest x-ray?
b Suggest six possible causes for such a lesion.

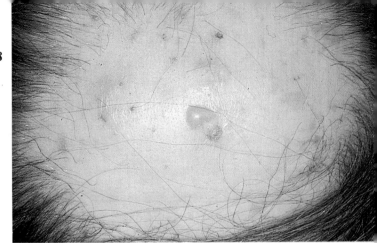

8 This patient is thyrotoxic and is about to undergo thyroid surgery. Over the past ten days he has developed an intensely pruritic eruption over his knees, elbows, buttocks and scalp. The scalp lesions are shown. There has been no response following benzyl benzoate applications, nor to topical steroid application.
a What is the diagnosis?
b What is the significance of impending thyroid surgery?

9 Extensive bruising developed after this child received an intramuscular injection. His platelet count, bleeding time and prothrombin time are normal, but activated partial thromboplastin time is prolonged.
a What is the most likely diagnosis?
b What is the chance that his younger brother will also suffer from this condition?

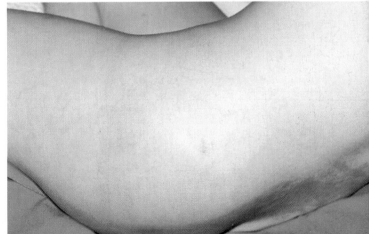

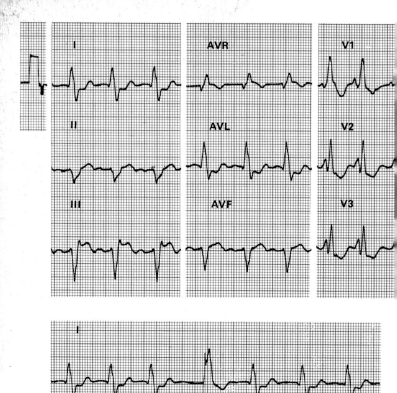

620 a What abnormalities does this ECG show?
   b What is the underlying diagnosis?
   c What treatment has been initiated?
   d Is he likely to require this therapy after discharge from hospital?

621 This sixty-two year old man complains of tiredness and nausea. He
   admits to excessive thirst, and to a tendency to constipation. His serum
   calcium is 2.96 mmol/l. Serum albumin is 34 g/l.
   a What principal abnormality is seen in this lateral abdominal x-ray?
   b What is the most likely diagnosis?
   c Would you recommend conservative management?

622 This patient suffers from migraine.
   a Which drug may have caused the abnormality shown?
   b How should this have been avoided?

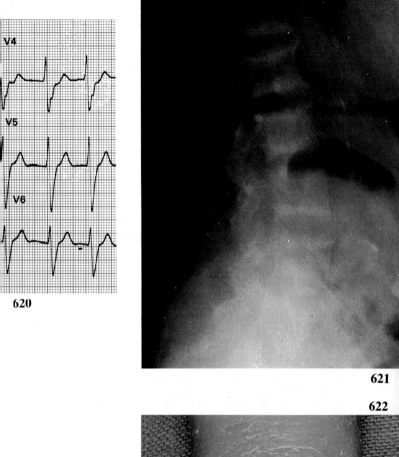

620

621

622

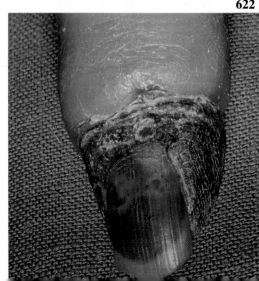

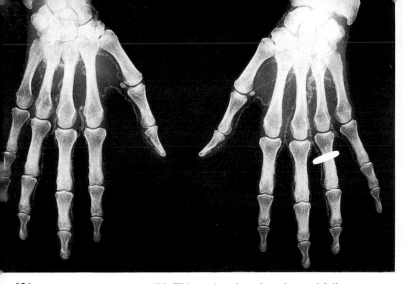

623

623 This patient has chronic renal failure.
What abnormalities are seen in the hands?

624

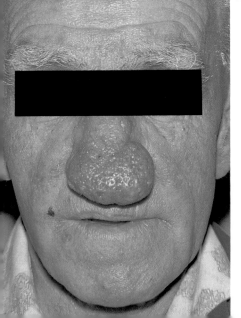

624 This patient has acne rosacea.
  a List five typical clinical features of uncomplicated rosacea.
  b What complication has developed?

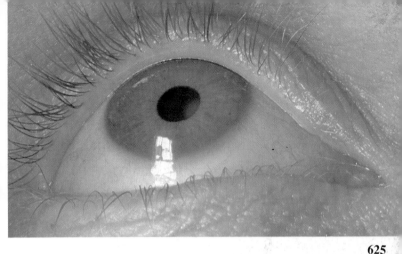

625

625 This young female patient complains of gradually progressive hearing loss.
    a What ocular abnormality is seen?
    b What cause of her hearing loss does this suggest?

626

626 This patient has psoriasis.
    a What treatment has he received?
    b What are the main complications of this form of therapy?

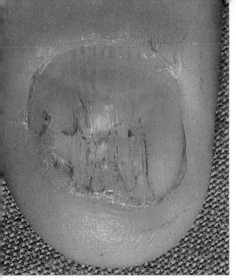

627

628

627 and 628

a What is the cause of the nail and penile abnormalities seen?

b What are the characteristic histological features of this condition?

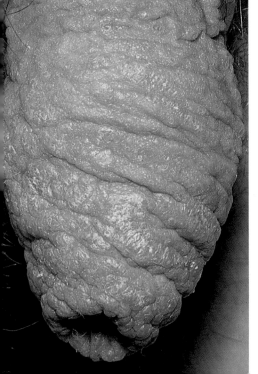

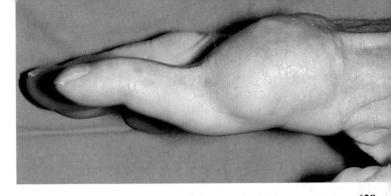

629 and 630 This patient has been aware of gradually enlarging painless lumps in his hands for some time. He has no joint symptoms.
   a What abnormalities are seen in the x-ray?
   b What is the most likely nature of the swellings?

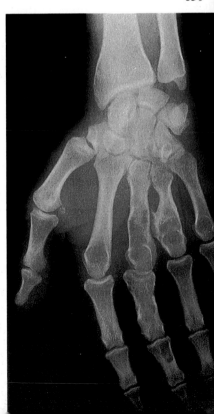

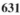

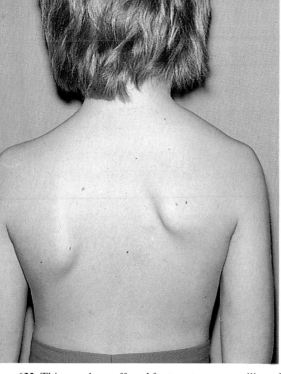

631

a Which is the
abnormal shoulder?
b What is the
deformity called?
c With which
condition may it be
associated?

632 This man has suffered from recurrent swelling of his face and arms, as
have several members of his family.
a What is the likely diagnosis?
b How should an acute attack be treated?
c What prophylactic therapy is available?
d What other symptom is common in this condition?

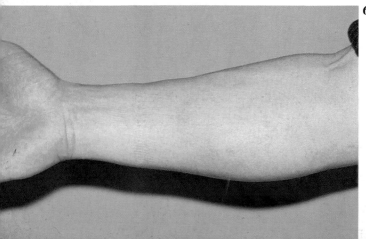

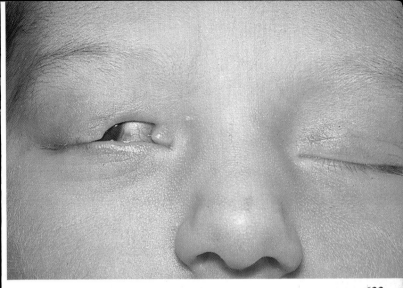

633

633 This lesion was present at birth.
    a What is it?
    b Is it associated with abnormalities of the iris?

634 a What abnormality is shown?
      b What important long term neurological complication may occur?

634

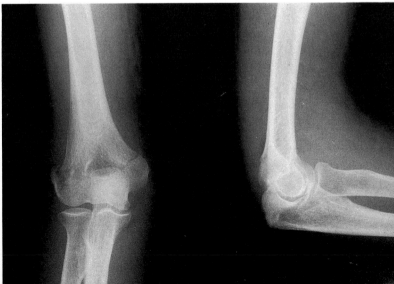

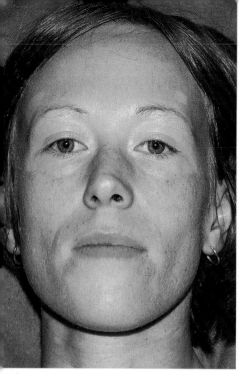

635 This twenty-eight year old woman presented with increasing tiredness. Her full blood count showed Hb 6.1 g/dl, WBC 3.1 x $10^9/1$, platelets 98 x $10^9/1$, and MCV 124 fl.
a What principal abnormality is shown?
b What is the likely diagnosis?

635

636 a Describe the abnormality.
b What is the diagnosis?

636

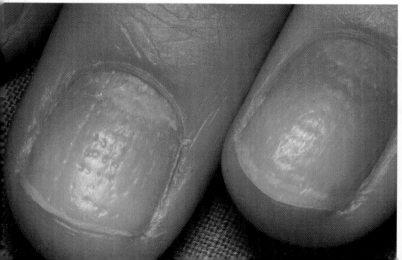

637
This goalkeeper complains of persistent pain in the hand dating from a punched goalmouth clearance during a recent football match.
What is the cause of his pain?

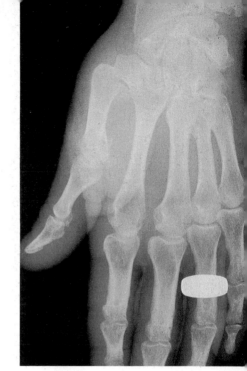

638
This patient has been blind in this eye since observing a solar eclipse without sunglasses several years ago.
a What is the cause of his blindness?
b What pupiliary abnormality would you expect to find?
c What precautions would have prevented his visual loss?

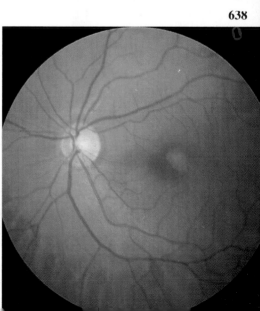

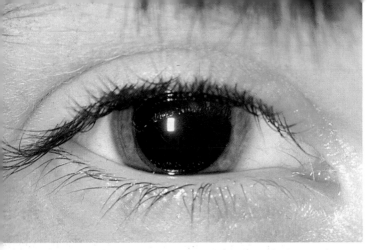

639

640

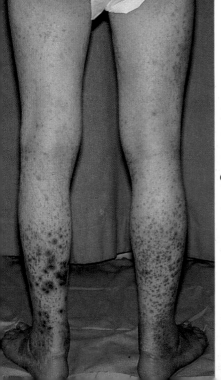

639 This girl has aortic regurgitation.
  a What ocular abnormality is demonstrated?
  b What is the diagnosis?
  c Will her daughters inherit this condition?

640 This man presented with haematuria and arthralgia following an acute upper respiratory infection.
  a What is the diagnosis?
  b Is this condition associated with streptococcal infection?
  c Which type of antibody is involved in this condition?
  d Is the bleeding time normal?

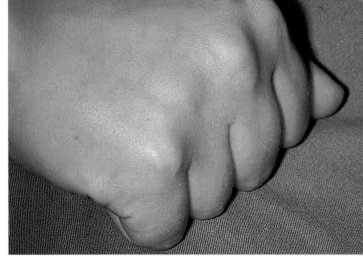

641 This man has mixed gonadal dysgenesis.
  a What abnormality is shown and in which other diseases may it occur?
  b What is his karyotype most likely to be?
  c Is he likely to be of normal stature?
  d What other external features may be present?

642 This is the fundus of a twenty-six year old man who presented with gradual loss of vision in his right eye.
  a What is this condition called?
  b What visual abnormalities may be detectable?

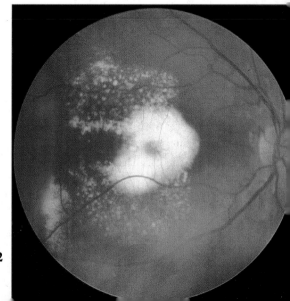

642

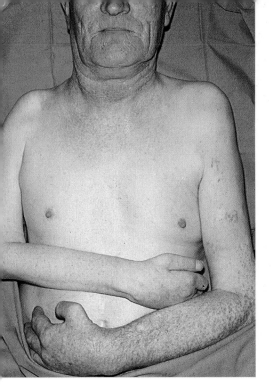

643

a What abnormalities are seen in this picture?

b Suggest three possible causes.

644

This twenty-four year old male patient complains of severe pain over the right shoulder and outer upper arm for ten days. There is no history of injury. He has been asked to push against the wall in front.

a What neurological abnormality is seen here?

b What is the likely diagnosis?

643

644

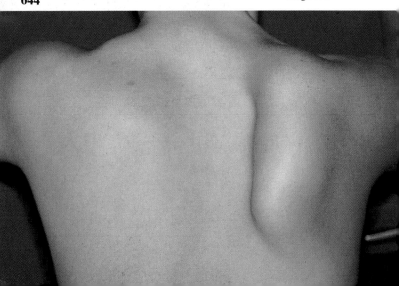

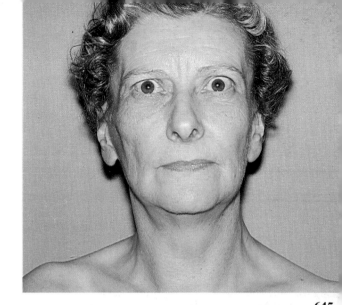

645

645 This patient has lost ten kilograms in weight over three months. She is on no regular medication.
  a What is the most likely diagnosis?
  b List four possible causes.

646

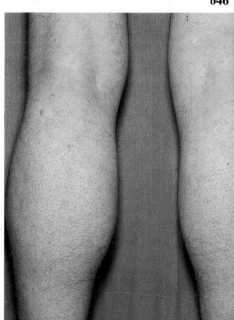

646 This sixteen year old boy first began to walk at the age of two. He has severe proximal muscle weakness in the legs with absent knee and ankle jerks.
  a What abnormality of the calves is seen?
  b What is
    i)   the likely diagnosis and
    ii) how is this disorder inherited?
  c List six other disorders which have the same mode of inheritance.

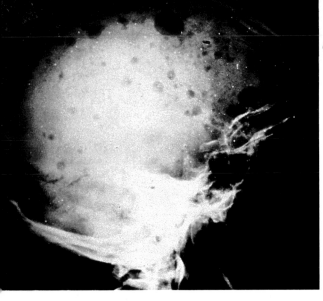

647

647 and 648 This patient presented with symptoms of hypercalcaemia.
  a What abnormalities are present
    i)   in the blood film?
    ii)   in the skull x-ray?
  b Which diagnosis does this suggest?
  c What change in alkaline phosphatase activity might be expected?

648

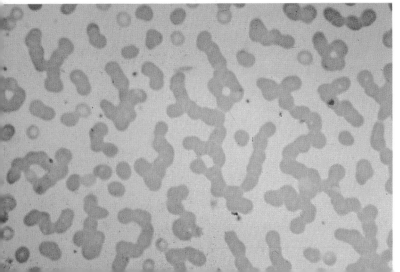

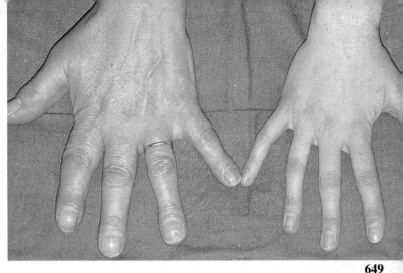

649

649 The hand on the left belongs to a woman who presented with bilateral carpal tunnel syndrome.
  a What is the diagnosis?
  b What is the effect on growth hormone secretion of administering thyrotrophin releasing hormone to such patients?
  c This disease may occasionally show a familial distribution. With which other conditions may it then be associated?

650

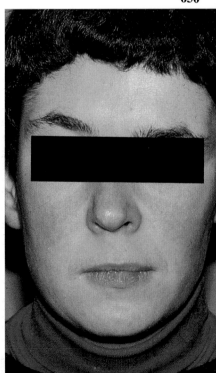

650 This anosmic woman presented with delayed puberty.
  a What facial abnormality is present?
  b Which diagnosis does this triad suggest?
  c What is the cause of her infertility?

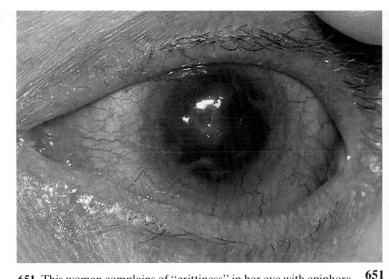

651 This woman complains of "grittiness" in her eye with epiphora, photophobia, and impaired vision.
  a What is the likely diagnosis and aetiology?
  b What specific therapies are available?

652 What abnormality is shown?

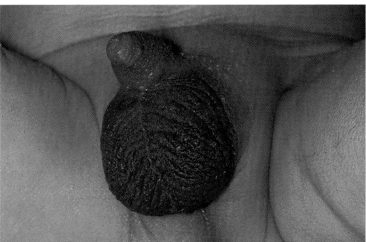

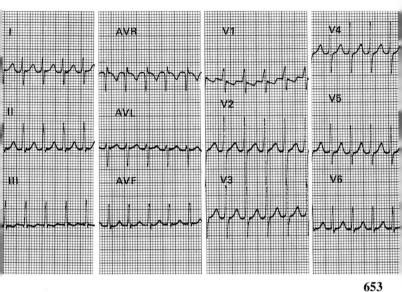

653

53 a What is this arrhythmia?
  b Name four physiological manoeuvres which may terminate this
     rhythm.
  c This patient became asystolic after being given intravenous verapamil.
     What treatment should be given?

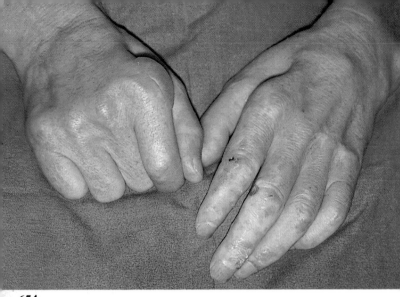

654

654 and 655 This man has normal touch sensation.
  a What abnormalities are shown?
  b Do these indicate a spinal level?
  c What further sensory testing should be performed?
  d If facial sensation is affected, will the corneal reflex be impaired?

655

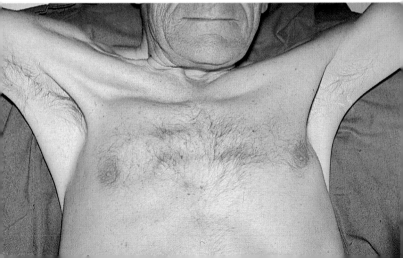

which area of the lung
this lesion?

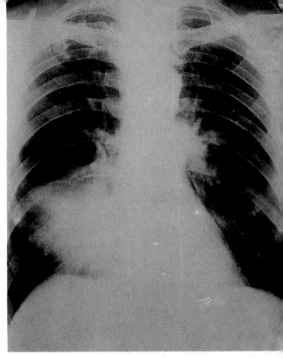

656

7 This woman has splenomegaly, peripheral neuropathy, heavy
proteinuria, and cardiac failure.
a What underlying diagnosis does this appearance suggest?
b In the secondary form of this disease, what is the commonest
associated condition
i) in the United Kingdom?
ii) worldwide? **657**

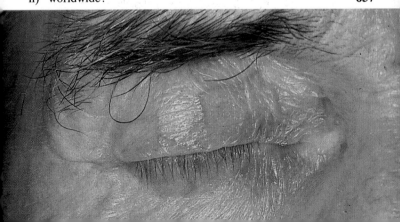

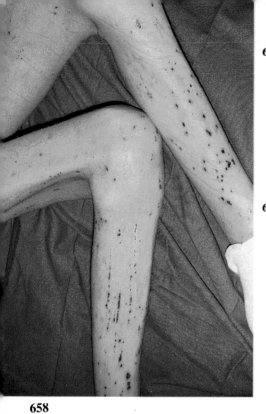

658 This patient has rapidly progressive liver disease. List three skin abnormalities seen and suggest an underlying cause for each.

659 This man presented with femoral fracture after falling out of bed. He was found to have hepatosplenomegaly. A full blood count showed pancytopaenia.
  a What conjunctival abnormality is demonstrated?
  b i) What is the underlying condition?
     ii) How is it acquired?
  c Is he likely to develop neurological consequences of this disease?

658

659

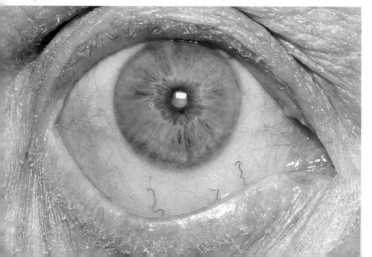

660 This woman presented
with a left calf deep
venous thrombosis. Prior
to commencement of
anticoagulants, her
Activated Partial
Thromboplastin Time was
found to be prolonged.
  a What is the underlying
     condition?
  b Explain the coagulation
     abnormality in
     association with the
     deep venous
     thrombosis.

661 This patient presented
with acute abdominal
pain. He was found to
have acute pancreatitis.
  a What complication has
     developed?
  b What biochemical
     abnormality may help
     establish the diagnosis?
  c Which investigations
     may confirm the
     diagnosis?

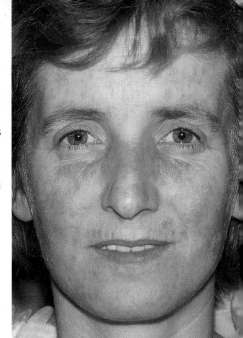

660

661

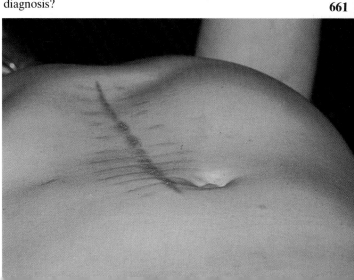

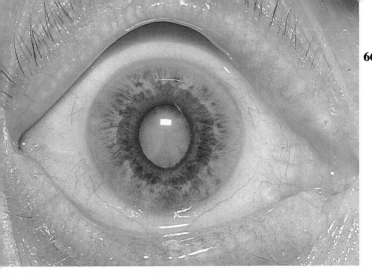

662

662 a What ocular abnormality is shown?
    b Would you expect this patient's visual acuity to improve on pinhole testing?

663 This patient has suddenly become hypotensive, tachypnoeic and centrally cyanosed. Arterial blood gas analysis reveals PCO_2 2.8 kPa, PO_2 5.4 kPa.
    a What principal abnormality is seen in the lung fields?
    b What is the likely diagnosis?
    c What immediate treament should be considered?

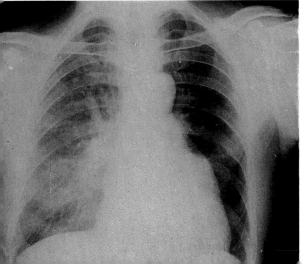

663

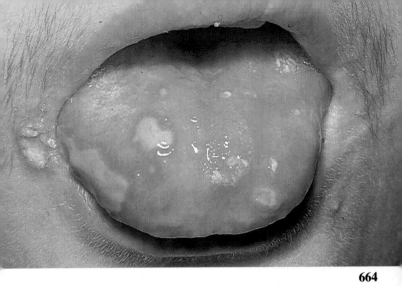

664

665

664 and 665 This patient
suffers from recurrent
genital and oral
ulceration. In an attempt
to corroborate the
suspected diagnosis,
saline was injected
intradermally into the
forearm. Culture of fluid
expressed from the lesion
produced no organisms.
a What is the likely
   diagnosis?
b What is the most
   typical ocular
   manifestation of this
   disorder?

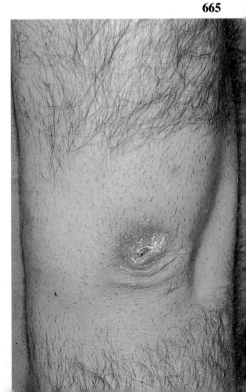

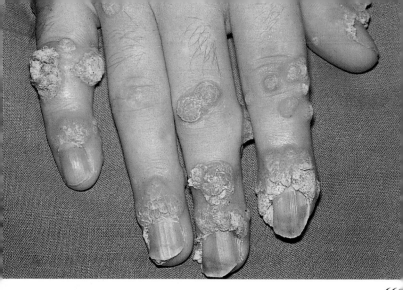

666 a What are these lesions?
    b What is the causative agent?
    c Which two underlying causes should be suspected here?

666

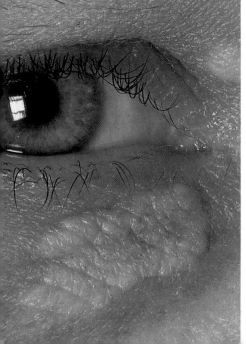

667 This patient is concerned about the cosmetic appearance of her eyelids.
    a What is the likely nature of the lesions seen?
    b What local therapy may be effective?

667

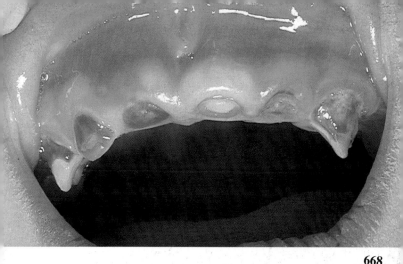

668

668 This two year old child's mother was given ampicillin for urinary infection during her pregnancy and tetracycline while she was breast feeding. The child's older brother has similar dental abnormalities. What is the likely cause of the dental abnormalities?

669

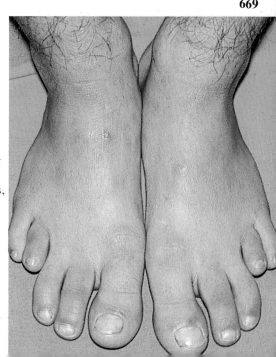

669

This patient complains of generalised muscle weakness, muscle cramps, and paraesthesiae of hands and feet. Chvostek's and Trousseau's signs are positive.

a What abnormality of his feet is seen?
b What diagnosis does this suggest?

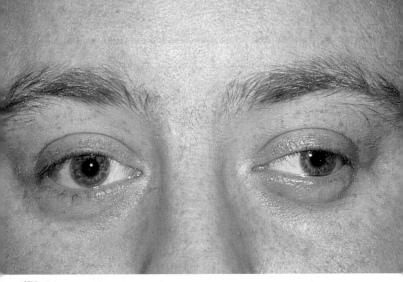

670

670 On lateral gaze this man develops nystagmus in the abducting eye. In this photograph, he has been asked to look to the left.
   a What abnormality is present?
   b What name is given to these features?
   c What is the anatomical site of the lesion and which disease is usually responsible?

671 a What abnormality is visible on this skull x-ray?
      b What is the likely diagnosis?
      c List six serious local complications of this condition.

671

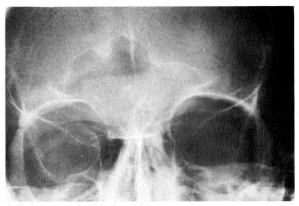

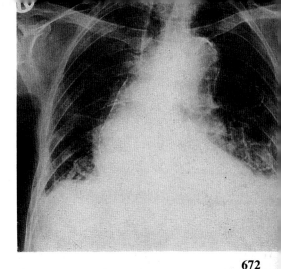

672

672 This patient has angina of effort which responds poorly to sublingual glyceryl trinitrate.
   a What principal abnormality is seen on the chest x-ray?
   b What is the diagnosis?
   c What is the cause of his angina?
   d What two abnormalities might be found on inspection of the trachea?

673

673
This patient suffers from a chronic inflammatory joint disorder. Routine biochemical analysis reveals a moderately raised serum alkaline phosphatase activity. Gamma glutamyl transferase (transpeptidase) activity is normal.
What is the most likely cause of the biochemical findings?

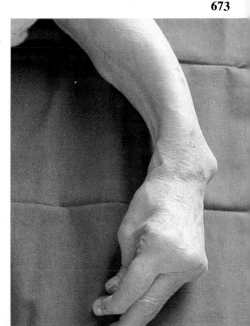

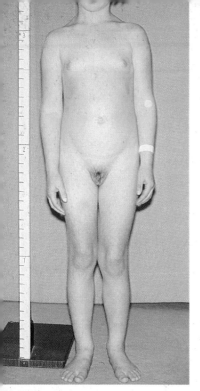

674 This five year old girl is
tallest in her class at
school.
a What abnormalities are
present?
b What is the diagnosis?
c State the possible
underlying disorders.

675 This x-ray was taken three
months ago when the
patient, a motorcyclist,
fell heavily from his
motorcycle. Although the
shoulder is now pain free
the patient still finds
difficulty in lifting the
arm.
a What abnormality is
seen on the x-ray?
b What complication of
this has occurred?
c What neurological
abnormalities would
you expect to find?

674
675

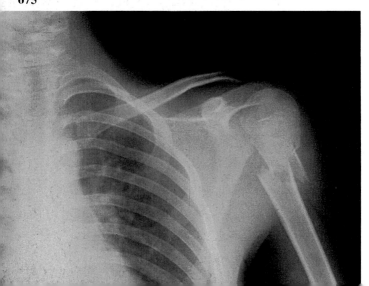

676

This patient has no visual symptoms, is normotensive and is not diabetic.

a What name is given to the lesions seen in the fundus?

b What is their pathological basis?

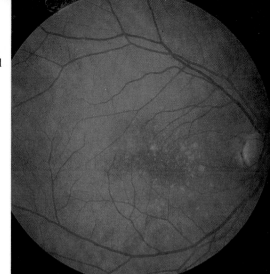

677

This is the knee of a sixteen year old haemophiliac boy.

a What condition has developed?

b What is the immediate treatment?

c Should the joint be routinely aspirated?

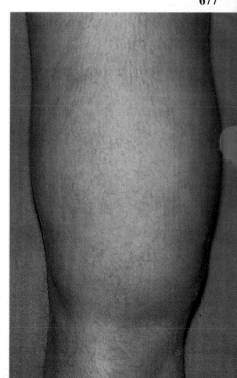

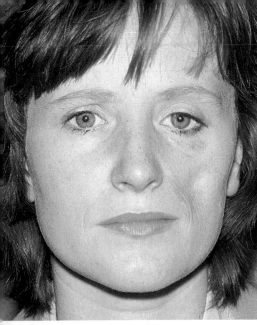

678
a What is this condition?
b At what age does it usually present?
c Is the right side of her face likely to become affected?

679
This twenty-six year old woman driver received head and facial injuries following a head-on collision with another vehicle. On admission to the Accident and Emergency ward she complained of central chest pain. She denied symptoms prior to the accident. Electrocardiogram showed T wave inversion across the chest leads. Over the next twenty-four hours there was a significant rise in serum creatinine kinase and aspartate aminotransferase activities. A diagnosis of myocardial infarction was made and she was transferred to the coronary care unit.
a What abnormality is seen on her lateral chest x-ray?
b What alternative diagnosis does this suggest?

678

679

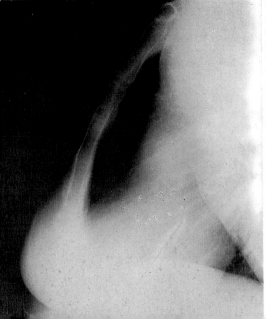

680 This patient has neutropenia, anaemia and thrombocytopenia. Bone marrow biopsy reveals hypocellularity of all cell series. Erythropoiesis is normoblastic.

a What is the likely cause of the swellings seen in the forearm?

b Suggest three possible causes of this patient's pancytopenia, related to the cause of the forearm lesions.

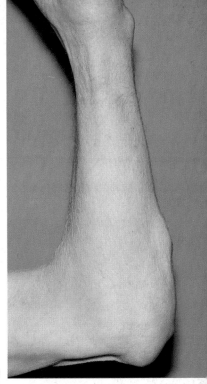

680

681 This patient has become hypotensive twenty-four hours after the onset of a diarrhoeal illness. She is drowsy and confused and is unable to give a history. Her plasma glucose on stick testing is 2 mmol/l.

a What diagnosis is suggested by the appearance of her mouth?

b How would you confirm this diagnosis biochemically without delaying replacement therapy?

681

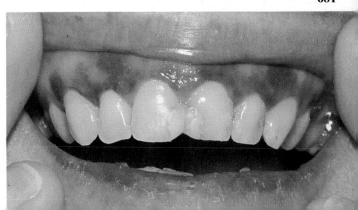

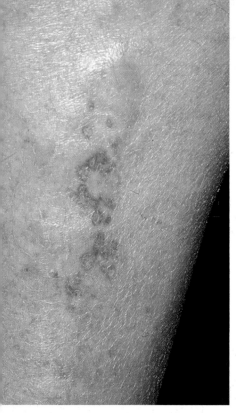

682

682 This obese patient suffers
from recurrent leg
ulceration which is slow to
heal.
a What is the most likely
cause?
b List five other skin
manifestations of this
disorder.

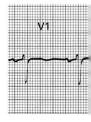

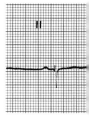

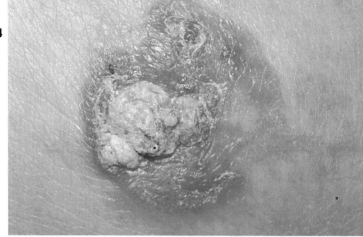

684 The lesion on this patient's breast has shown no improvement after a week of topical corticosteroid therapy.
a What is the diagnosis?
b What is its significance?

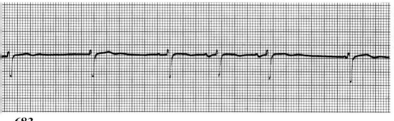

683

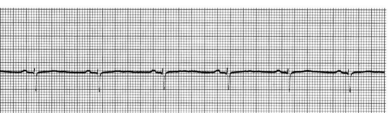

683 This seventy year old man presented with recurrent syncopal episodes. Examination was completely normal.
a What abnormality is present? (The traces are not synchronous).
b What is the likely diagnosis?
c What further investigation is likely to be of value?

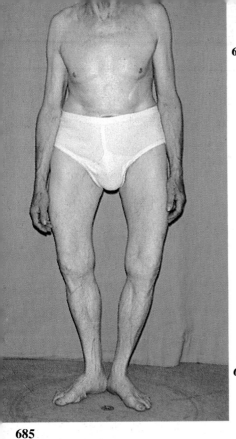

685 a What is this disease?
b What is the basic cellular abnormality?
c What is the risk of malignant change?

685

686 a With which conditions is this appearance associated?
b Is further investigation indicated?
c Is there an increased risk of low back pain in patients with this appearance?

686

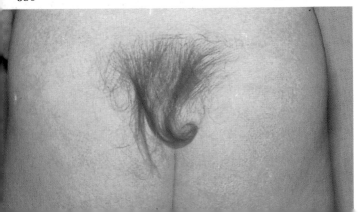

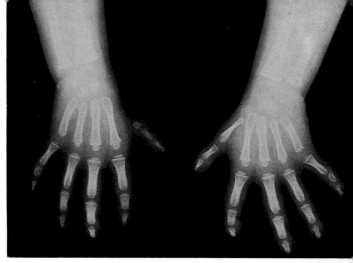

687 This boy has a pancytopaenia noted since birth.
  a What abnormality is present?
  b What is the diagnosis?
  c What ocular abnormality may be present?

688 This child was brought to his practitioner's attention by the health visitor
  who suspected non-accidental injury.
  a What is this lesion?
  b With which haematological abnormalities may it be associated?

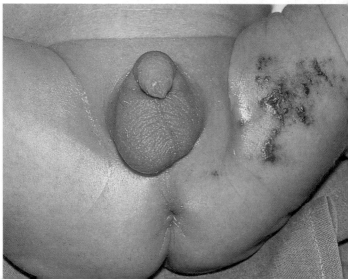

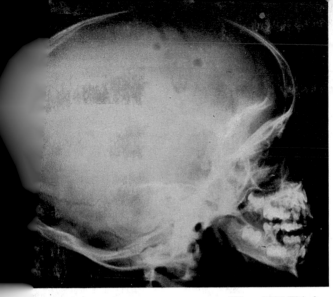

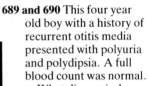

689

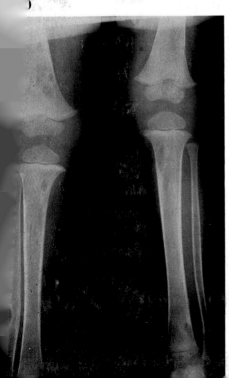

689 and 690 This four year
old boy with a history of
recurrent otitis media
presented with polyuria
and polydipsia. A full
blood count was normal.
a What diagnosis does
   this appearance
   suggest?
b What is the cause of his
   polyuria?
c What is the prognosis?

691 This thirty year old man complains of coldness and tingling in the feet. He suffers from recurrent superficial thrombophlebitis of the calves and feet?

    a What is the likely diagnosis?

    b Which other feature of the history is important in corroborating this diagnosis?

    c His radial arterial pulses are absent. Does this modify your diagnosis?

692 This child was unconscious for a minute after she fell from the branch of a tree. She now complains of having a runny nose.

    a What abnormalities are seen here?

    b What is the diagnosis and what complication may have occurred which would explain the new symptom?

    c What treatment is indicated?

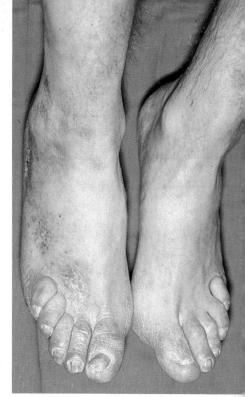

691

692

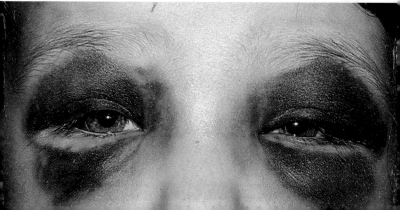

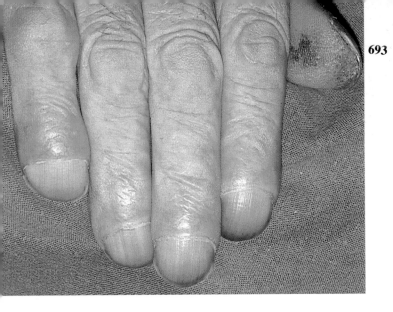

693

693 and 694 This elderly patient complains of pain in the wrists at night.
a What is the principal radiological abnormality?
b What is the cause of his symptoms?
c What is the most likely underlying diagnosis?

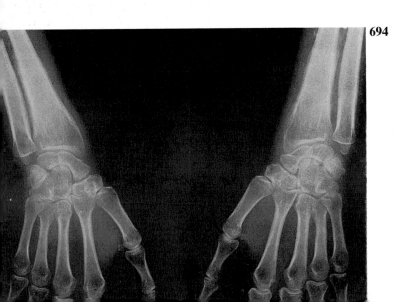

694

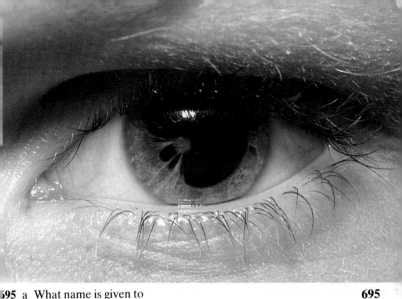

695 a What name is given to
the abnormalities seen
in this patient's eye?

b What past ocular
disorder do they
indicate?

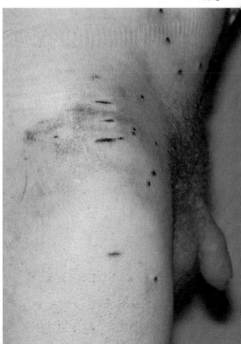

695

696

696 a What cause is
suggested by the
morphology and
distribution of the
lesions seen on this
patient's thigh and
abdomen?

b Are these lesions likely
to have been self-
inflicted?

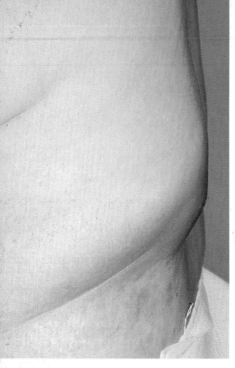

697 This woman gives a seven day history of rigors and severe pain and swelling in her left flank. She has also experienced recent urinary frequency, dysuria and one episode of haematuria.

a What is the likely diagnosis?

b What underlying renal disease may give rise to this condition?

c What may her chest x-ray show?

697

698 This patient complains of chronic pain above her ankle. The pain is usually worse at night.

a What is the diagnosis?

b What is the likely aetiology?

698

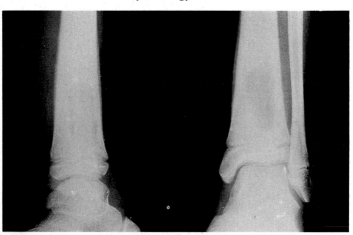

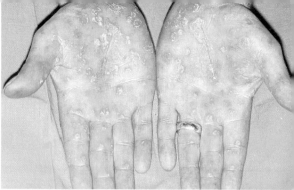

699

700

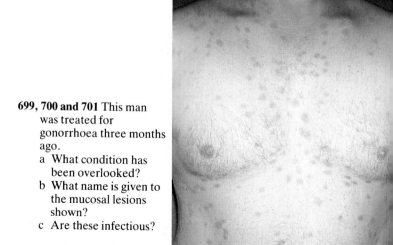

701

699, 700 and 701 This man
was treated for
gonorrhoea three months
ago.
a What condition has
been overlooked?
b What name is given to
the mucosal lesions
shown?
c Are these infectious?

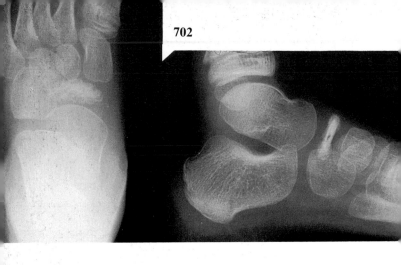

702 and 703 These are related conditions.
  a What are the diagnoses?
  b What is the underlying pathophysiology?
  c Are these patients likely to develop long term complications?

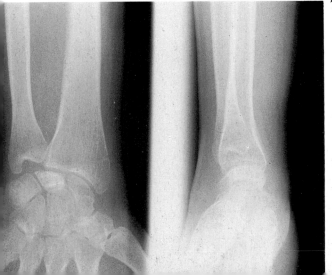

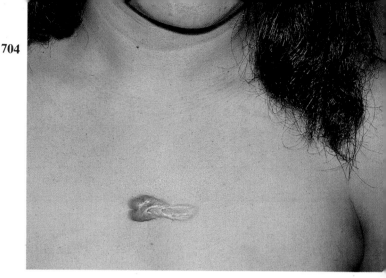

704 a What is this lesion?
b What groups of patients are at risk of developing this condition?

705 This woman had a corneal ulcer which was treated with topical steroids.
a What complication has developed?
b Which three organisms are usually responsible?

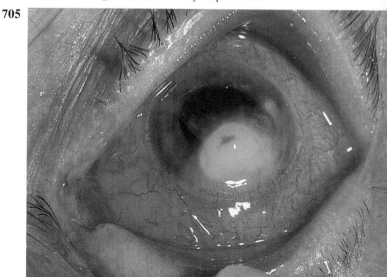

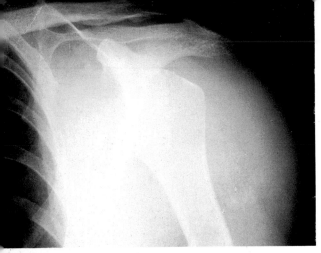

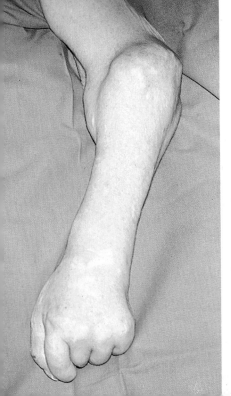

706 and 707 This patient has been aware of painless limitation of movement of the left elbow for several years. The x-ray was taken after a recent fall onto the left shoulder.

a What name is given to the type of joint abnormalities seen?

b Suggest three possible diagnoses.

c What is the cause of the lesions seen on the skin of hand and forearm?

708

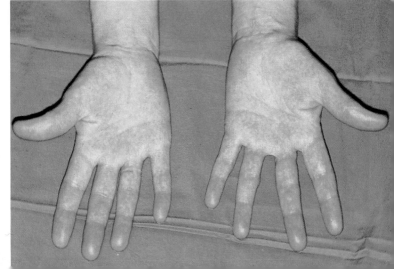

708
This diabetic man
complains of marked
proximal muscle
weakness and pain as well
as dysaesthesiae over the
anterior aspect of his
thighs.
a What abnormality is
   seen in the illustration?
b What is the diagnosis?
c How would you treat
   this disorder?

709 a Describe the abnormality seen in these hands.
     b What endocrine disorder is typically associated with these
       appearances?
     c List five other dermatological manifestations of this disorder.

709

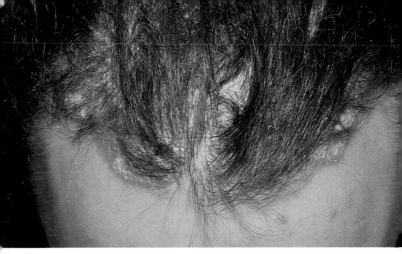

710

711

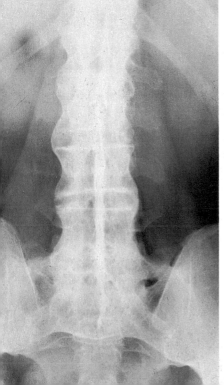

710 and 711 This patient complains of stiffness in his back and hips. He has no ocular symptoms. A cursory examination of the skin of limbs and trunk reveals no abnormalities.

a What abnormality is seen on x-ray of lumbar spine?

b What diagnosis is suggested by the appearance of the hairline?

c Which other areas of skin should be examined closely for evidence of this condition?

712 a What is this
investigation?
b What does it show?
c Which transmissable
fungal agent
characteristically
induces these
appearances?
d What abnormalities
would you expect on
skin testing?

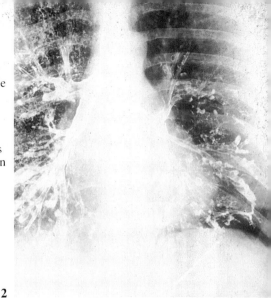

712

713 This man had a partial gastrectomy five years ago for an antral gastric
ulcer. His haemoglobin is 9.8 g/dl and mean corpuscular volume 82 fl.
a What two abnormalities are present?
b What is their aetiology?
c What simple investigation is indicated?

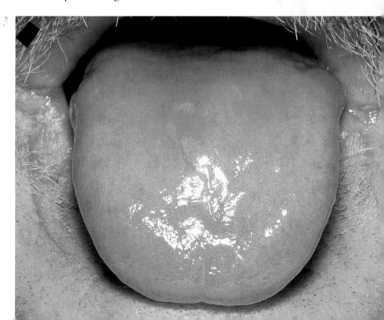

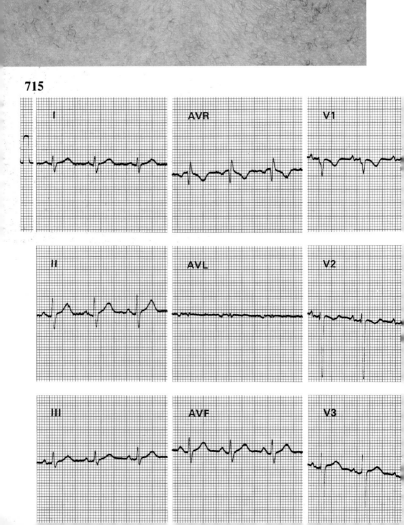

714

715

714 and 716 This elderly bachelor has been admitted to hospital after a fall at home. Forty years ago an acute duodenal ulcer was managed medically; there have been no exacerbations in the past twenty years. He has a mild macrocytic, normochromic anaemia.

a What principal abnormalities are seen of
   i)   his abdominal skin?
   ii) his legs?
b What is the likely cause?

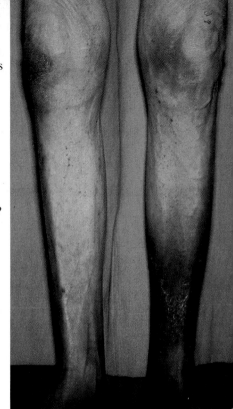

716

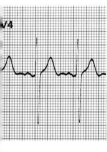

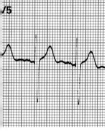

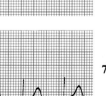

715 a What name is given to this pattern?
b With which conditions is it associated?

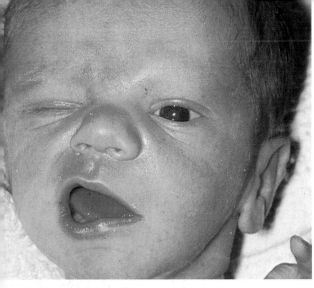

717 a Why is this baby
winking?
b Which iatrogenic factor
may be involved in the
aetiology of this
condition?
c What is the likelihood
of recovery?

718

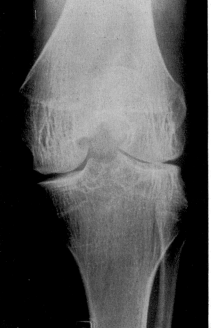

718 a What is the principal
abnormality seen in this
young patient's knee?
b Which inherited
disorder typically
produces this
appearance?

719 The abnormality seen in this twenty-two year old patient's hand persists when the arm is elevated, and has been present for several months.
  a What is the diagnosis?
  b Suggest two possible causes.

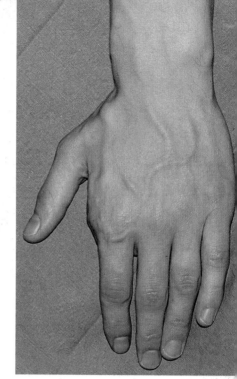

719

720 a What is this condition?
  b In which two ways do the associated visceral lesions typically present?

720

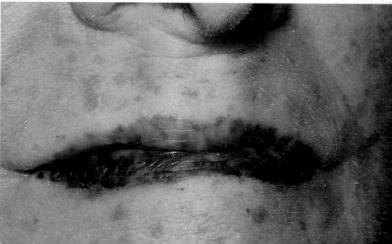

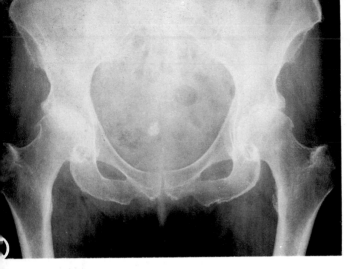

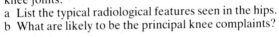

721 and 722 The same pathological process affects this patient's hip and
knee joints.
a List the typical radiological features seen in the hips.
b What are likely to be the principal knee complaints?

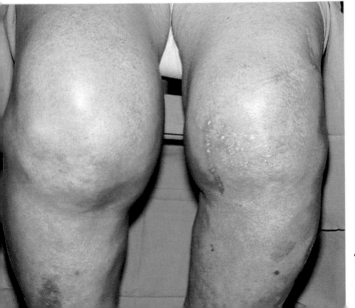

723 This patient complains of an itchy rash of several weeks duration. The larger darker lesion seen over the right scapula appeared before the rash became more widespread.
  a What name is given to this darker lesion?
  b What is the most likely cause of this rash?

724 This patient has longstanding rheumatoid arthritis. He has been admitted to a general surgical ward following the sudden onset of severe central abdominal pain. There is generalised abdominal tenderness, guarding and rigidity. Bowel sounds are absent.
  a What pathological process underlies the skin lesions seen?
  b Suggest four possible causes of his current illness relating to the underlying disease or its management.

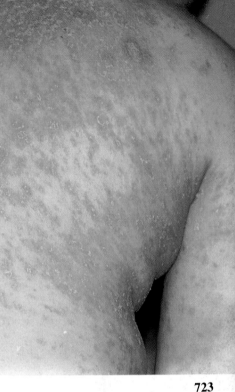

723

724

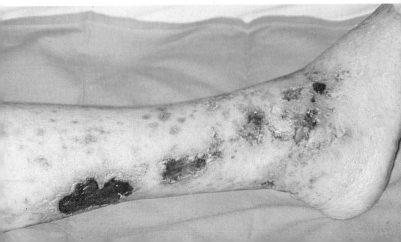

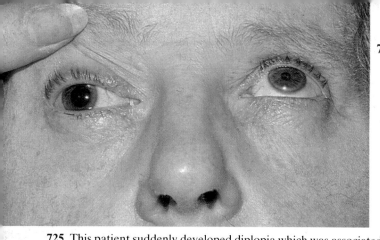

725 This patient suddenly developed diplopia which was associated with left-sided clumsiness and incoordination. She has been asked to look upwards.
  a What abnormality is present?
  b Where is the underlying lesion situated and which structures are involved?
  c Which eponymous name is given to this condition?

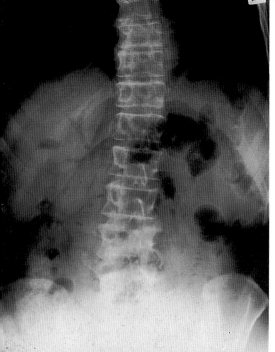

726
This woman complained of vomiting and right upper quadrant abdominal pain. This settled initially but after 48 hours, she developed further vomiting, abdominal distension and obstructive bowel sounds. An initial abdominal x-ray was normal.
  a What abnormalities are present on this abdominal film?
  b What is the most likely diagnosis?
  c Would you expect the underlying cause to be visible on an x-ray?

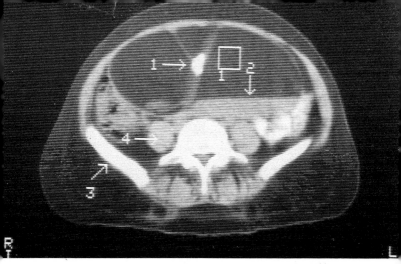

27 This is a CT section through the lower abdomen of a fifty-one year old nun who presented with generalised abdominal distension that had progressed over several years.
  a Name the structures 1 to 4.
  b A region of interest (ROI) is labelled as box 1, giving a density reading of −92.9 CT units. What tissue is this?

28 This girl claims to have ingested paraquat.
  a Does her appearance substantiate this claim?
  b Of what does her immediate management consist?
  c Should pulmonary fibrosis occur, which treatment may offer benefit?

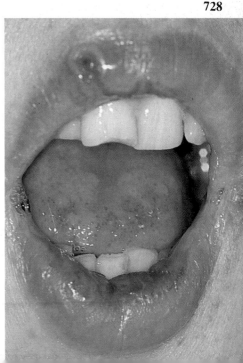

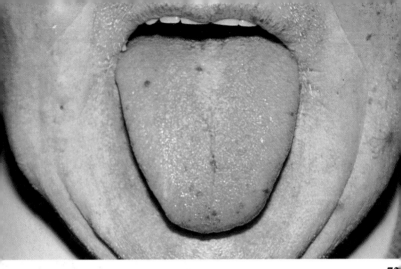

729 This patient presented with haemoptysis.
  a What physical sign should be sought?
  b What is the diagnosis?

730

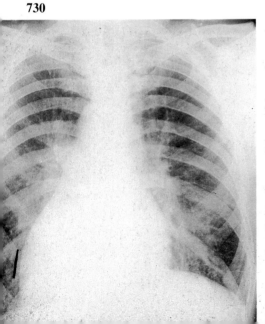

730
This patient has become acutely dyspnoeic.
a List four abnormalities seen in this posteroanterior chest x-ray.
b ECG shows sinus rhythm and biphasic P waves in lead V_1. What type of drug is your first choice in management?

731 This patient complains of intense nocturnal pruritus.
   a What diagnosis should be considered?
   b How is this best established?
   c What are the principles of treatment?

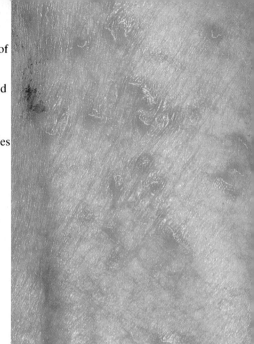

731

732

732
a What condition is this?
b List four possible underlying conditions.
c What is the principal complication?

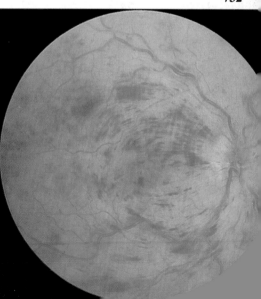

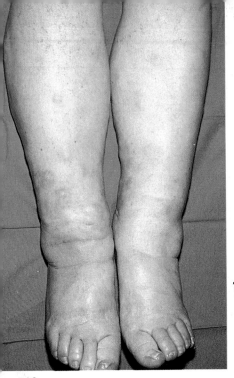

733 and 734

  a What abnormalities are seen in this patient's eyes and legs?

  b What is the diagnosis?

  c Which two other clinical features complete this syndrome?

733

734

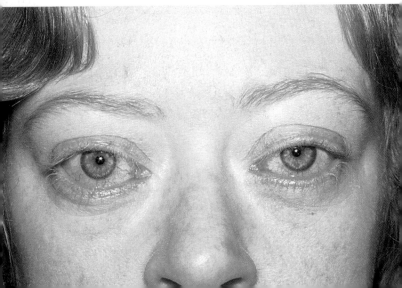

735 a What is the cause of
 this appearance?
 b What name is given to
 this condition?
 c Which ossicles may be
 involved?

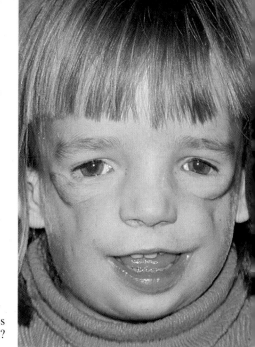

735

736 a What abnormality does
 this x-ray demonstrate?
 b What symptoms may
 the patient have?
 c What will passive
 movements of the arm
 show?

736

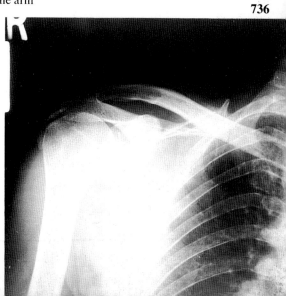

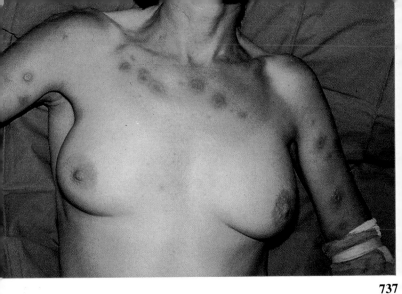

737

737 and 738
  a What abnormalities are seen on
      i) the skin?
      ii) the chest x-ray?
  b How may these conditions be associated?

738

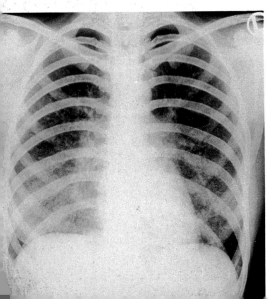

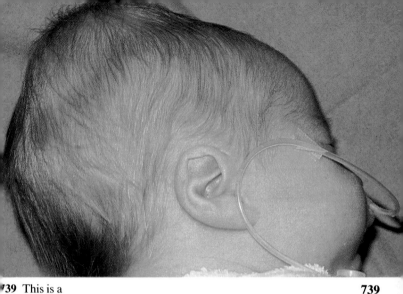

739 This is a
cephalhaematoma.
  a Where are such lesions
     situated in the scalp
     and what form the
     boundaries?
  b How can this be
     differentiated from a
     caput succedaneum?
  c Should routine
     aspiration be
     performed?

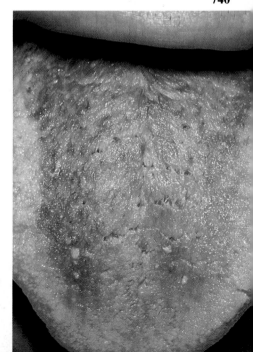

740 a What is this condition
          and what is the
          aetiology?
       b With which factors may
          it be associated?
       c How may it be treated?

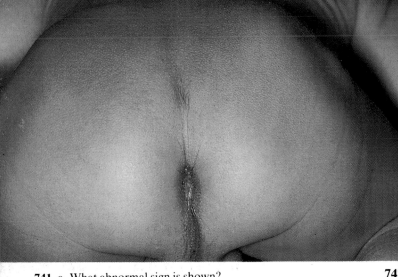

741 a What abnormal sign is shown?

74

b What will x-rays of the lumbosacral spine show?

742 This elderly patient has no visual complaints.

a What principal abnormality is seen in the optic fundus?

b What is the likely diagnosis?

c What measurement is indicated?

d What abnormality of this would you expect to find?

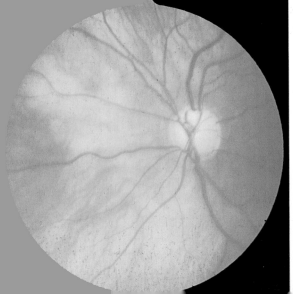

742

743 This obese patient complains of painful lumps over his abdomen, and of diffuse joint pains for the past two weeks. In addition to the skin abnormality, abdominal examination reveals shifting dullness.
  a What is the likely cause of the skin lesions?
  b This condition is associated with underlying disease of which abdominal organ?

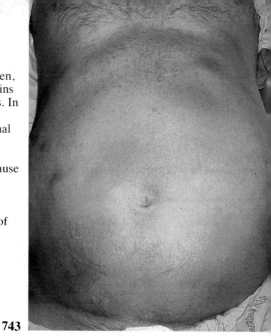

743

744 This patient has a six month history of a dense right hemiplegia. Two days ago she complained of pain in the right calf.
What condition has now developed?

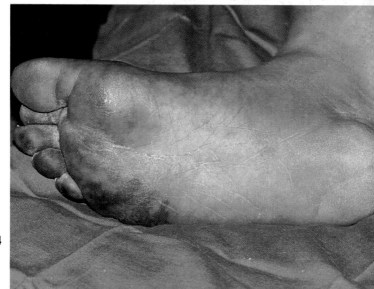

744

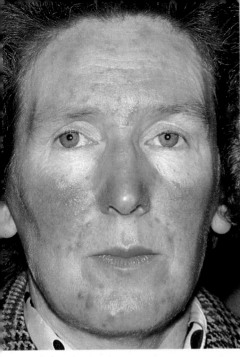

745 This patient complains of recurrent facial flushing, and of persistent facial redness.
a What is the most likely cause of her facial appearance?
b Suggest four conditions which may cause a similar appearance.

745

746 This child complains of generalised pruritus. The skin lesions seen are present on the forearms and thighs.
a What diagnosis is suggested by their appearance?
b How is this confirmed?

746

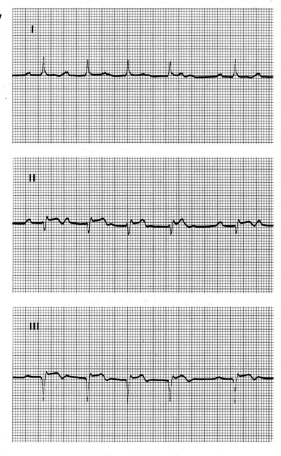

I

II

III

747 a What abnormality does this rhythm strip show?
   b What is the likely underlying cause?
   c Is this dysrhythmia always pathological?

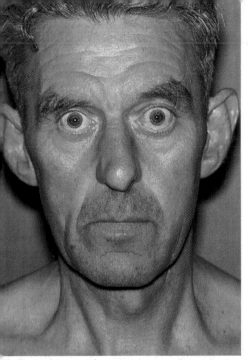

748 This man complains of weight loss and muscle weakness. Examination confirms marked proximal myopathy with no sensory loss.
  a Which differential diagnoses should be considered?
  b What clinical features shown here allow you to make the correct diagnoses?
  c How would you confirm this diagnosis?
  d How should this man be treated?

748

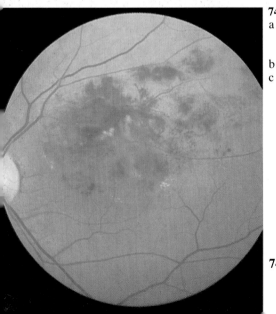

749
  a What abnormalities are seen in this patient's left eye?
  b What is the diagnosis?
  c What is the prognosis for intact central vision?

749

750 What are the causes of this tongue abnormality?

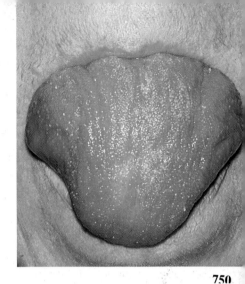

750

751

751 This man has chronic lymphocytic leukaemia.
  a What complication has developed?
  b What form of immunodeficiency is present?
  c How might this be confirmed at the bedside?

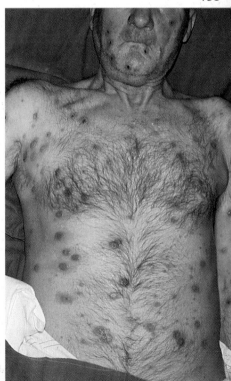

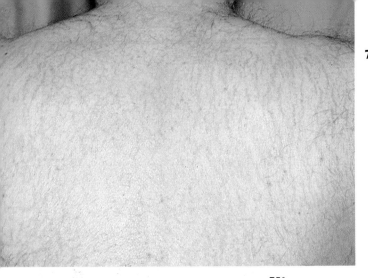

752

752
This man presented with an extensive non-pruritic eruption.
a What name is given to this appearance?
b With which conditions may this appearance be associated?

753

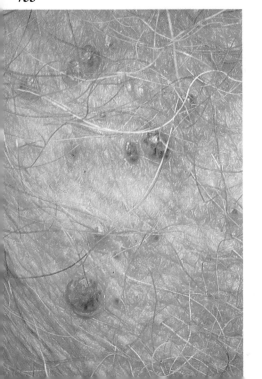

753
This twenty-eight year old male homosexual has recently noticed these lesions on his scrotum; there are no similar lesions elsewhere. Biopsy shows ectasia of the dermal vessels, with hyperkeratosis of the overlying epidermis.
a What is the likely diagnosis?
b What abnormality of his peripheral white cell count would you expect?

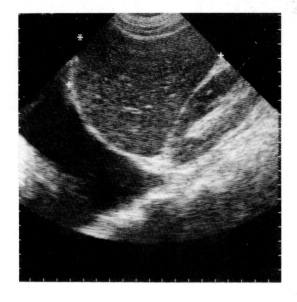

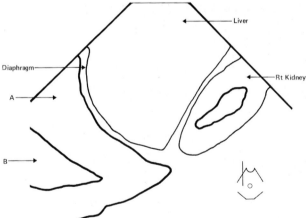

754 This sixty year old woman who had pelvic surgery one year ago now presents with breathlessness. This para-sagittal scan through the right lobe of the liver shows no abdominal abnormality.
 a Name the features labelled 'A' and 'B'.
 b Suggest the probable reason for her initial surgery.

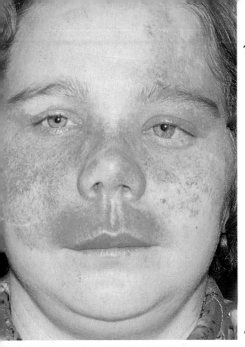

755 This girl has epilepsy.
  a Which syndrome is likely?
  b In which two other sites do similar lesions typically occur?
  c What may be seen on skull x-ray?

755

756 a What abnormality is seen on this chest x-ray?
  b Which three auscultatory signs are typical of this condition?

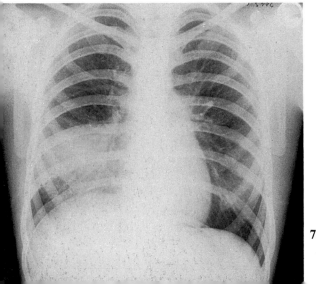

756

757 a What abnormalities are shown in this nine year old boy?
  b Name the condition.
  c What is the earliest sign of puberty in male children?

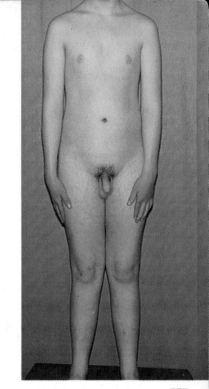

758 a What is the cause of the appearance of this optic fundus?
  b What other forms of treatment are available for this type of eye disease?

757

758

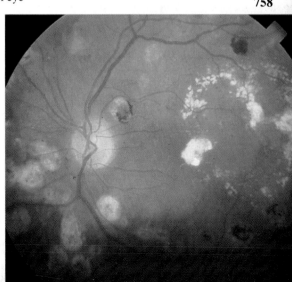

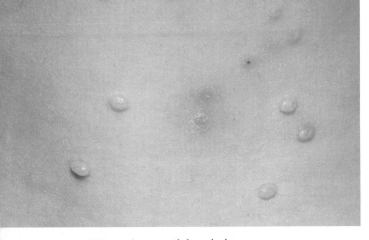

759 This child's mother noted these lesions.
   a What is the diagnosis?
   b What treatments are available?

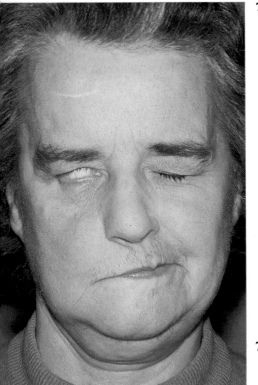

760 a What has this patient been asked to do?
   b What is this eye sign called?
   c Where does the affected cranial nerve exit from the skull?

760

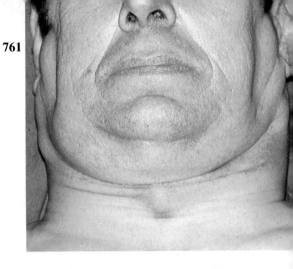

761 and 762 This man complained of swelling of his neck and axillae and of night sweats. Splenomegaly (5 cm) was noted. Node biopsy showed Hodgkin's lymphoma.
a What clinical stage is his disease?
b What therapy is appropriate?
c What are the histological criteria of this disease?

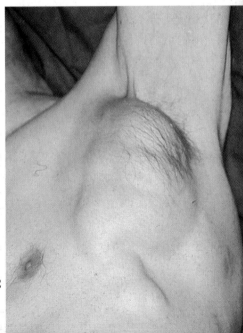

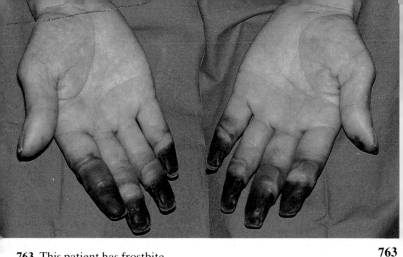

763 This patient has frostbite.   **763**
Would you recommend rapid active rewarming or slow passive
rewarming?

764 This woman complained of severe headache then collapsed.
Examination revealed a flaccid left hemiplegia, subhyaloid fundal
haemorrhages, blood pressure of 230/140mm Hg and pulse rate of 48 per
minute.
a What is the cause of her collapse?
b Should her blood pressure be reduced immediately?

764

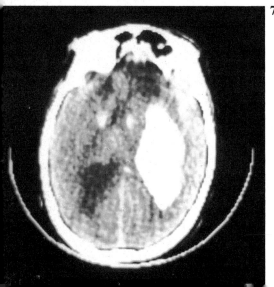

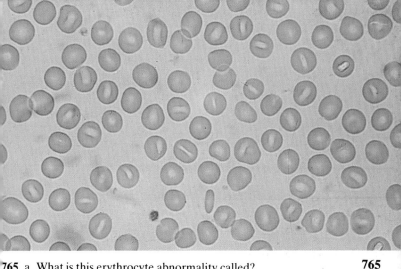

765 a What is this erythrocyte abnormality called?
   b With which conditions is it associated?
   c What is the underlying cellular defect?

765

766 This patient has been involved in a road traffic accident.
   a List three abnormalities visible on the chest x-ray.
   b What is the hydrostatic pressure in a normal pleural space?

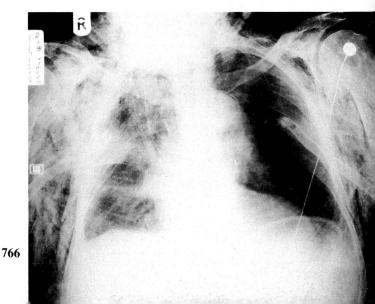

766

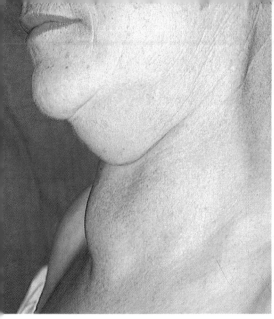

767

This woman presented with menorrhagia.
a What abnormality is present?
b What is the likely diagnosis?
c What is the likely aetiology of this condition?

767

768 This patient has rheumatoid arthritis, and complains of severe pain in this eye.
a What is this condition?
b What is the principal ocular complication?

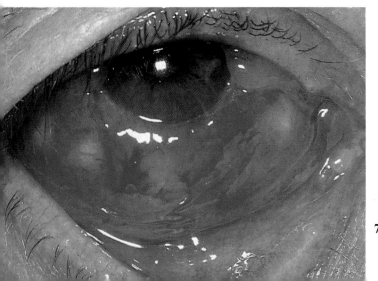

768

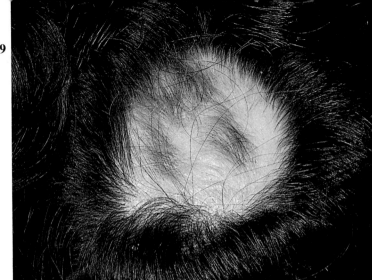

769 This patient complains of a patch of baldness on her scalp. Close examination reveals 'exclamation mark' hairs at the edges of the bald patch. She has no skin rash, but nail pitting and thickening are observed.
a What is the most likely diagnosis?
b What is the likelihood that the hair will regrow within a year?

770 This is the hand of a forty-five year old woman.
a What is the cause of this appearance?
b What are the likely causes?

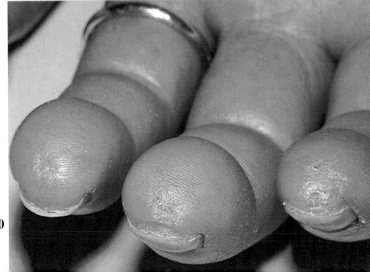

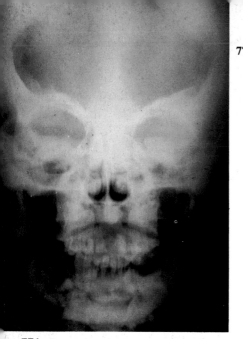

771

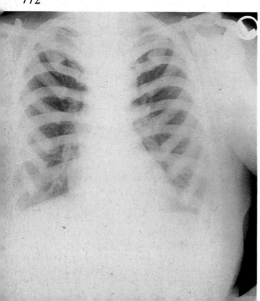

772

771 and 772 This patient complains of increasing deafness for several months, and more recently of exertional dyspnoea and tiredness. A year ago a wrist fracture required twelve weeks in plaster. Haematological results include: Hb 9.2 g/dl; white cell count 1.5 x $10^9/1$: differential count, — neutrophils 48%, lymphocytes 30%, myelocytes 4%, metamyelocytes 4%; Nucleated red cells also seen.

a What is the diagnosis?
b What is the mode of inheritance of this condition?
c Which bone is typically spared?
d What treatment is available?

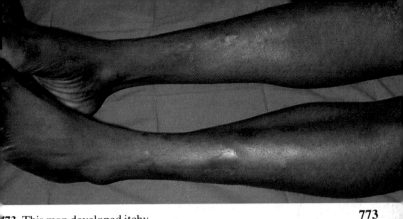

773 This man developed itchy papillomatous lesions over his shins which healed with scarring during childhood. Shortly after this, a widespread maculopapular eruption appeared followed by desquamation. His VDRL and TPHA tests are both positive.
  a Which non-venereal infection can explain all these findings?
  b Which single serological test will differentiate this from syphilis?

773

774

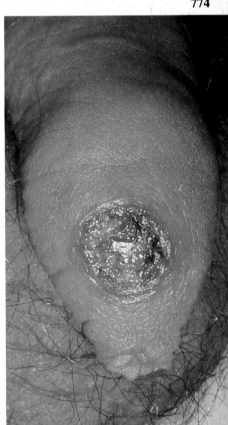

774 This patient presented with this painless lesion.
  a What is the most likely diagnosis?
  b How is this confirmed?
  c Which serological test becomes positive first?

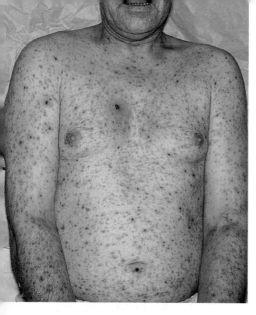

775 and 776 This man has acute myeloid leukaemia.
Which two infections has he developed?

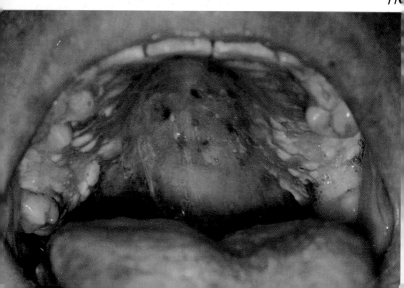

ANSWERS

The answers given below are necessarily brief as the aim of the series is to stimulate self-learning through further reading.

583 a Leishmania tropica.
b Phlebotomine sandflies.
c No.
d Yes, with the development of cell-mediated immunity and a delayed skin (leishmanin) reaction.

584 i) Phenytoin administration with associated poor oral hygiene.
ii) Scurvy.
iii) Acute myeloid leukaemia.

585 and 586
a Distended superficial veins. Blood flow caudally is demonstrated.
b Superior vena caval obstruction.
(Portal hypertension is not the cause here. The veins on the left side of the abdomen are seen not to extend radially from the umbilicus).

587 a 1 Right ventricle.
2 Aorta.
3 Left ventricle.
4 Inter ventricular septum — grossly enlarged.
5 Left atrium.
6 Mitral valve papillary muscles.
b Hypertrophic cardiomyopathy. Gross hypertrophy of inter ventricular septum is causing obliteration of the left ventricular cavity in systole.

588 a Herpes virus hominis, type II.
b Meningitis associated with primary infection.

589 a Koebner phenomenon.
b Lichen planus, eczema.

590 a i) Perioral bruising.
ii) Pallor.
b i) Bleeding tendency with anaemia secondary to blood loss.
ii) Combined anaemia and thrombocytopenia secondary to primary marrow failure, or to peripheral destruction/sequestration of red cells and platelets.

591 a To obtain instruction about a gluten free diet in respect of dermatitis herpetiformis.

b IgA, often in the dimeric form.

592 a Ectropion.

b Age-related loss of muscular tone in the lower lid.

593 a Massive pericardial effusion and right pleural effusion.

b i) Pulsus paradoxus; hypotension.

ii) An elevated JVP, rising on inspiration (Kussmaul's sign).

594 a Microfilaria (of Loa loa).

b i) Lymphatic filariasis (Bancroftian and Malayan).

ii) Loiasis.

Others include infection with Dipetalonema perstans and Mansonella ozzardi.

Microfilaria of Onchocerca volvulus are not seen in the peripheral blood.

c Eosinophilia.

595 a Localised hyperostosis of the skull vault.

b Meningioma.

596 a Diffuse reticulonodular shadowing.

b i) Restrictive ventilatory defect: low forced expiratory volume in one second (FEV_1) and forced vital capacity (FVC). (Ratio of FEV_1 to FVC may be normal.) Diminished lung volumes (Residual volume and total lung capacity).

Reduced transfer factor.

Diminished lung compliance.

ii) Arterial hypoxaemia, more pronounced on exercise. Normal or low normal pCO_2.

597 Drug overdose — eg. barbiturates
                             tricyclic antidepressants

Carbon monoxide poisoning.

598 a Galactorrhea.

b Hyperprolactinaemia.

c i) Dopamine receptor blockers eg. phenothiazines, butyrophenones, metoclopramide and others like pimozide, sulpiride.

ii) Catecholamine depleting agents eg. reserpine, methyl dopa.

iii) Others — oestrogens; narcotics.

599 a Orf.

b A pox virus.

c Sheep farming. (Veterinary surgeons, sheep shearers are also at risk

00 a i) Streptococcal tonsillitis/pharyngitis.
  ii) Infectious mononucleosis (glandular fever).
 b i) Throat swabs — film for Gram staining and bacteriological culture.
  ii) Antistreptolysin 0 titre.
  iii) Infectious mononucleosis slide or monospot tests; Paul Bunnell test.
  iv) Blood film — looking for atypical mononuclear cells.

01 a Achondroplasia.
 b Autosomal dominant.
 c Cephalopelvic disproportion is likely
   — baby's head is large
   — pelvic deformity if mother is achondroplastic.

02 a 'Mooned' face, facial plethora, hirsutism.
 b Cushing's syndrome.
 c Plasma adrenocorticotrophic hormone assay.

03 a Rubeosis iridis, suffused conjunctiva, oval pupil (impaired red reflex).
 b Acute glaucoma.

04 a i) Thyroglossal cyst.
  ii) Thyroid nodule.
 b i) Ask the patient to swallow — a thyroid nodule will rise in the neck.
  ii) Ask the patient to protrude her tongue — a thyroglossal cyst will rise. (Thyroglossal cyst may also be fluctuant, and may transilluminate).

05 a Conjunctival haemorrhage.
 b Whooping cough (but may occur in most respiratory illnesses associated with prolonged coughing episodes).
 c Bordetella pertussis (a Gram negative aerobic coccobacillus).

06 a Optic atrophy.
 b Retrobulbar neuritis.

07 a Lanugo hair.
 b Anorexia nervosa.

08 a Acromegaly.
 b i) Overproduction — Growth hormone.
      — Prolactin.
      — Thyroid stimulating hormone (T.S.H.) which can lead to T.S.H. dependent hyperthyroidism.

    ii)   Deficiency   — Adrenocorticotrophic hormone (A.C.T.H.)
                           — T.S.H.
                           — Luteinising hormone (L.H.).
                           — Follicle-stimulating hormone (F.S.H.).
                           — Vasopressin.
    iii)   Antagonism   — of insulin action by growth hormone.
                                 (hyperinsulinaemia in some).

609 a Chronic tophaceous gouty arthritis.
      b Hyperuricaemia.
      c i)   Frequent attacks of acute gout (eg > 4/year).
         ii)   Renal disease.
         iii)   Young patients with raised serum uric acid and family history of
               cardiac or renal disease.
         iv)   Excessive purine production (syndromes of increased purine
               synthesis eg. Lesch-Nyhan, and increased turnover eg.
               lymphoproliferative disorders [especially if chemotherapy
               used].)
         v)   Tophaceous gout.

610 a i)   Hirsutism — excessive hair growth on face and chin.
         ii)   Acne.
      b i)   Ovarian — polycystic ovary syndrome; androgen producing
               tumours eg. arrhenoblastoma, hilar-cell tumour etc.
         ii)   Adrenal — congenital adrenal hyperplasia, including partial
               defects; adrenal hyperplasia, adrenal adenoma and carcinoma.
         iii)   Idiopathic hirsutism.
         iv)   Hyperprolactinaemia.
         v)   Drugs — Androgens, phenytoin.

611 a Necrobiosis lipoidica diabeticorum.
      b Diabetes mellitus.

612 Squamous carcinoma of skin. Multiple arsenical keratoses.

613 a Group A beta-haemolytic streptococcus.
      b Yes. The eponym is St. Anthony's fire.

614 Skin necrosis as a result of radiotherapy following mastectomy for
     carcinoma of breast.

615 a Cryptogenic fibrosing alveolitis.
      b No, the risk is increased.

616 a Erythema gyratum repens.
      b Associated with underlying malignancy (especially bronchus, breast)

17 a 'Coin' lesion in the right lower zone.
b Differential diagnosis includes
  i)   Bronchogenic or alveolar cell carcinoma.
  ii)   Secondary tumour ('cannonball' secondary).
  iii) Hamartoma.
  iv)   Arteriovenous malformation.
  v)   Rheumatoid nodule.
  vi)   Tuberculosis.
  vii) Chondroma (of chest wall).
  viii) Encysted pleural effusion.

18 a Dermatitis herpetiformis.
b This condition is aggravated by potassium iodide (used in rendering patients euthyroid prior to surgery).

19 a Haemophilia A (factor VIII deficiency).
b Usually sex linked recessive (although occasionally arises by spontaneous mutation) — risk therefore depends on whether mother is carrier or haemophiliac (rare). Father's genotype is irrelevant.
If mother carrier, risk is 1 in 2.
If mother haemophiliac, all sons will be affected.

20 a First degree heart block with left axis deviation; complete right bundle branch block; ST elevation in leads II, III and AVF with reciprocal ST depression in leads I and AVL; a single paced complex.
b Acute inferior myocardial infarction.
c A right ventricular pacemaker has been inserted.
d No. Permanent pacemaker insertion more commonly follows anterior myocardial infarction.

21 a Nephrocalcinosis.
b Primary hyperparathyroidism.
c No. Nephrocalcinosis is regarded as an indication for parathyroid surgery.

22 a Ergotamine.
b By restricting its use to acute migrainous attacks. Ergotamine should not be used prophylactically.

23 i) Arterial calcification.
    ii) Subperiosteal erosions.

24 a i) Erythema.
      ii) Telangiectasia.
      iii) Swelling.
      iv) Papules.
      v)   Pustules.
b Rhinophyma.

625 a Blue sclera.
    b Otosclerosis (in association with osteogenesis imperfecta tarda — typ
      1 osteogenesis imperfecta).

626 a PUVA (Psoralen, Ultra Violet A).
    b i)   Sunburn.
      ii) Exacerbation of psoriasis.
      iii) Herpes simplex infection.
      iv) Potential risks (not yet defined) —
           ocular solar burns
           accelerated skin ageing
           malignancy — skin (especially melanoma), haematological.

627 and 628
    a Lichen planus.
    b i)   Epidermal cell degeneration (formation of 'colloid bodies').
      ii) Liquefaction necrosis of the basal cell layer.
      iii) Subepidermal lymphocytic infiltrate.
      iv) 'Saw tooth' appearance of the rete pegs.

629 and 630
    a Lytic areas with expansion of the medullae, in a number of
      metacarpals and phalanges.
    b Enchondromata.
      (Although there is swan neck deformity of the right index finger, this
      is not rheumatoid disease).

631 a The right.
    b Sprengel's shoulder.
    c Klippel-Feil syndrome (congenital fusion of cervical vertebrae with
      resulting short neck and low hairline).

632 a Hereditary angioedema.
    b Patency of the airway must be maintained. Fresh frozen plasma will
      restore C1 Esterase inhibitor activity. Adrenaline, hydrocortisone,
      and antihistamines are usually given but have little effect. Aprotinin
      and epsilon-aminocaproic acid (EACA)may also be employed.
    c Danazol is the most effective prophylaxis. Avoidance of trauma is
      important. Surgery can be covered with fresh frozen plasma.
      Testosterone and EACA may also be used.
    d Recurrent abdominal pain.

633 a Coloboma of eyelid.
    b No.

634 a Supracondylar fracture of humerus.
    b Ulnar nerve paralysis

635 a Perioral and periocular vitiligo.
    b Pernicious anaemia.

36 a Nail pitting.
    b Psoriasis.

37 Fracture of base of 1st metacarpal (Bennett's fracture).

38 a Solar burn.
    b None.
    c Indirect observation (that is of the sun's image projected onto black
       surface through a pinhole). Sunglasses (and exposed photographic
       film) do not reliably protect the eye.

39 a Dislocation of the lens upwards.
    b Marfan's syndrome.
    c 50% of them are likely to be affected.

40 a Henoch-Schonlein purpura.
    b Yes.
    c IgA.
    d Yes.

41 a Short fourth metacarpal, which may be found in Turner's syndrome,
       pseudohypoparathyroidism and pseudo-pseudohypoparathyroidism.
    b 45XO/46XY mosaicism.
    c No.
    d The somatic features of Turner's syndrome.

42 a Coat's disease (It is a central exudative reaction occurring in young
       men and of unknown aetiology).
    b Reduced visual acuity; central scotoma.

43 a Shortening of the right arm (especially of the upper arm); wasting of
       right shoulder and arm.
    b i)   Childhood paralytic poliomyelitis.
       ii) Brachial plexus injury in childhood.
       iii) Cerebral palsy.

44 a Winged right scapula.
    b Neuralgic amyotrophy (brachial neuritis).

45 a Hyperthyroidism.
    b i)   Graves' disease — diffuse toxic goitre.
       ii) Toxic nodular goitre — single adenoma, multinodular, thyroid
           carcinoma (well differentiated, but usually with metastases).
       iii) Subacute or chronic thyroiditis.
       iv) Factitious (self-administration of thyroxine).
       v) Secondary to thyroid stimulating (TSH) hormone overproduction
          — functioning pituitary adenoma.
       vi) Ovarian teratoma (struma ovarii) (iv, v and vi are rare causes).

646 a Pseudohypertrophy.

  b i) Duchenne muscular dystrophy. (Becker's dystrophy is unlikely with such an early onset).

   ii) Sex linked recessive.

  c These include
   i) Red-green colour blindness.
   ii) Haemophilia A; Haemophilia B (Christmas disease).
   iii) Glucose-6-phosphate dehydrogenase deficiency.
   iv) Bruton's agammaglobulinaemia.
   v) Angiokeratoma corporis diffusum (Fabry's disease).
   vi) Testicular feminisation syndrome.
   vii) Chronic granulomatous disease.
   viii) Lesch-Nyhan syndrome.

647 and 648

  a i) Rouleaux formation.
   ii) Multiple, well defined lytic lesions.

  b Multiple myeloma.

  c None; alkaline phosphatase activity is characteristically normal or only slightly elevated in multiple myeloma.

649 a Acromegaly.

  b Release of growth hormone occurs.

  c It may be associated with hyperplasia or adenomas of the parathyroids, pancreatic islets, adrenal cortex, and thyroid (multiple endocrine neoplasia syndrome, type I or Wermer's syndrome).

650 a Facial asymmetry secondary to hypoplasia of the left maxilla.

  b Hypogonadotrophic hypogonadism (Kallman's syndrome).

  c Failure of gonadotrophin secretion due to inadequate secretion of gonadotrophic releasing hormone from the hypothalamus.

651 a Dendritic corneal ulcer due to herpes simplex virus type 1.

  b 5-iododeoxyuridine, acyclovir, vidarabine, triflurothymidine, corticosteroids (only if the corneal stroma is involved).

652 None. This is a negro baby.

653 a Supraventricular tachycardia.

  b Carotid sinus massage, Valsalva maneouvre, ocular massage, application of cold water or ice-packs to the face or drinking iced water may stimulate a diving reflex.

  c Intravenous calcium; external cardiac massage and ventilatory support; insertion of a temporary pacemaker if rhythm is not quickly established.

654 and 655

    a Muscle wasting of the hands and sternocostal heads of pectoralis major; trophic changes in the fingers of the left hand; a large bulla on the base of the right index finger.

    b The sparing of the clavicular head of pectoralis major indicates a lesion below C6.

    c Pain and temperature testing must be performed. The patient has syringomyelia.

    d No. The corneal reflex is not mediated through the spinal tract of the trigeminal nerve.

656 The middle lobe of the right lung. There is loss of the right cardiac border unlike lower lobe lesions where the silhouette is preserved.

657 a Primary amyloidosis. Cutaneous involvement is less common in secondary amyloidosis.

    b i)   Rheumatoid arthritis.

      ii) Leprosy.

658 i) Jaundice — retention of bilirubin.

    ii) and iii) Haemorrhagic excoriations and purpura — pruritus secondary to bile salt retention; haemostatic failure secondary to

        — clotting factor deficiencies

        — thrombocytopenia

        — impaired clearance of fibrinolysins.

659 a Pingueculae.

    b i) Gaucher's disease, adult type.

      ii) Autosomal recessive.

    c No.

660 a Systemic lupus erythematosus.

    b The Activated partial thromboplastin time is prolonged due to a circulating anticoagulant, the lupus anticoagulant.

661 a Pancreatic pseudocyst.

    b Persistently elevated serum amylase.

    c Abdominal ultrasonography or computerised tomography are the most useful investigations.

662 a Absent red reflex: mature cataract.

    b No.

663 a Oligaemic left lung field.

    b Major pulmonary embolism (occluding right main pulmonary artery).

    c i) Heparin.

      ii) Thrombolytic agent (eg streptokinase).

      iii) Pulmonary embolectomy.

664 and 665
   a Behçet's disease.
   b Iridocyclitis (often with hypopyon).
   . Conjunctivitis, choroiditis and optic neuritis may occur.

666 a Common warts.
   b Human wart viruses (a group of papovaviruses).
   c i) Local trauma (especially nailbiting).
     ii) Impaired cell-mediated immunity (eg chronic lymphatic leukaemia).

667 a Xanthelasmata.
   b Trichloracetic acid.

668 Ectodermal dysplasia (a sex-linked inherited disorder).
   — Ampicillin in pregnancy has not been associated with dental abnormalities.
   — Tetracycline is chelated in breast milk: dental abnormalities are not associated with its use in these circumstances.

669 a Short fourth and fifth metatarsals.
   b Pseudohypoparathyroidism.

670 a Impaired adduction of the right eye.
   b Internuclear ophthalmoplegia with ataxic nystagmus.
   c Medial longitudinal fasciculus in the mid-brain; multiple sclerosis.

671 a Fluid level in the frontal sinus.
   b Frontal sinusitis.
   c i)   Cranial osteomyelitis.
     ii) Cavernous sinus thrombosis.
     iii) Meningitis.
     iv) Cerebral abscess.
     v)   Subdural empyema.
     vi) Extradural abscess.

672 a Calcification in an aneurysmal ascending aorta, and aortic arch. (There is also a left pleural effusion).
   b Syphilitic aortitis (acquired — aortitis is not a feature of congenital syphilis).
   c Combination of coronary ostial stenosis and ventricular hypertrophy (There may be concomitant coronary artery disease).
   d i) Tracheal deviation, to right.
     ii) Tracheal tug (i.e. descent in time with the heart beat).

673 Coexistent Paget's disease of bone. The picture shows sabre-like deformity of the radius, consistent with Paget's. Rheumatoid changes i the hand are also shown.

674 a Increased linear growth, development of oestrogen-dependent secondary sexual characteristics — developing breasts, development of pubic hair.

b Precocious puberty or precocious pseudopuberty.

c Precocious puberty —
  i) Idiopathic premature activation of hypothalamic pituitary function.
  ii) Central nervous system tumour.
  iii) McCune Albright syndrome.
  iv) (Hypothyroidism).

Precocious pseudopuberty —
  i) Factitious — exogenous oestrogens.
  ii) Ovarian tumours.
  iii) Adrenal tumour or congenital adrenal hyperplasia.

675 a Fracture of the surgical neck of the humerus.

b Axillary nerve damage.

c i) Weakness of deltoid (with difficulty in maintaining abduction of the arm; the nerve also supplies teres minor).
  ii) Sensory loss over the humeral insertion of the deltoid.

676 a Drusen (these are indistinguishable from exudates).

b Proliferative changes in the basement membrane of the pigment epithelium (Bruch's membrane) — degenerative.

677 a Haemarthrosis.

b Intravenous factor VIII; resting of the affected limb; analgesia if required.

c No, particularly if there is a factor VIII inhibitor.

678 a Facial hemiatrophy.

b During the second decade.

c No.

679 a Fractured sternum.

b Myocardial contusion, secondary to blunt chest injury.

680 a Rheumatoid nodules.

b i) Gold.
  ii) Penicillamine.
  iii) Phenylbutazone (This drug is no longer used in the management of rheumatoid disease in the U.K.).
  iv) Immunosuppressive drugs — cyclophosphamide, azathioprine.

Felty's syndrome (rheumatoid arthritis, splenomegaly, neutropenia or pancytopenia) is unlikely in the presence of a hypocellular marrow.

681 a Primary adrenal insufficiency.
  b i) Carry out a 'short Synacthen (corticotrophin) test.
      — Take plasma for baseline cortisol assay; give 25 IU Synacthen depot (corticotrophin), by intramuscular injection; repeat cortisol assay thirty minutes later.
    ii) Give dexamethasone or betamethasone as corticosteroid replacement initially (these will not interfere with plasma cortisol assay, unlike hydrocortisone or cortisone).

682 a Venous insufficiency.
    These include:
  b i) Varicose eczema.
    ii) Dependent oedema.
    iii) Chronic lymphoedema (often with skin hypertrophy).
    iv) Red cell extravasation/haemosiderin deposition.
    v) Secondary infection of ulcers/cellulitis.
    vi) White atrophy (atrophie blanche).(Malignant change in varicose ulcers is rare).

683 a Sinus arrest with idionodal escape rhythm.
  b Sick sinus syndrome.
  c Continuous ambulatory electrocardiographic (Holter) monitoring.

684 a Paget's disease of the nipple.
  b Accompanies intraduct carcinoma of breast.

685 a Paget's disease of bone.
  b Excessive osteoclastic bone resorption.
  c Sarcoma occurs in less than 1% of affected patients.

686 a Spina bifida occulta; diastematomyelia.
  b No. unless there are neurological symptoms or signs.
  c No.

687 a Hypoplasia of the thumbs.
  b Congenital aplastic anaemia (Fanconi's anaemia).
  c Strabismus.

688 a A cavernous haemangioma.
  b Thrombocytopaenia; hypofibrinogenaemia; elevated fibrin degradation products (Kasabach-Merritt syndrome).

689 and 690
  a Multifocal eosinophilic granuloma (Hand-Schuller-Christian disease)
  b Cranial diabetes insipidus.
  c Good. Recovery may occur spontaneously through chemotherapy or radiotherapy may be indicated for local disease. Diabetes insipidus may be permanent.

1 a Buerger's disease (thromboangiitis obliterans).
  b History of heavy cigarette smoking.
  c No. The radial pulses may be absent in 40% of cases.

2 a i) Superficial abrasions around right eye, bruising right scalp
        (external signs of the head injury).
    ii) Bilateral periorbital haematomata.
    iii) Right conjunctival haemorrhage.
  b Basal skull fracture: complicated by dural tear and cerebrospinal fluid
    (CSF) leak.
  c Prophylactic antibiotic(s) — eg penicillin and sulphadimidine.
    She should be admitted to hospital for observation. Surgical repair
    may be necessary if CSF rhinorrhoea persists.

3 and 694
  a Periosteal reaction along the radii.
  b Hypertrophic pulmonary osteoarthropathy.
  c Bronchogenic carcinoma.

5 a Posterior synechiae.
  b Iritis (anterior uveitis).

6 a Shotgun pellet wounds.
  b No. The scatter of pellet wounds indicates a point of discharge
    approximately ten metres from the subject. (Spread of lesions in cm.
    usually 2½-3 times range in metres).

7 a Perinephric abscess.
  b Pyelonephritis, usually associated with renal calculi.
  c Ipsilateral pneumonia, collapse, pleural effusion, or elevated hemi-
    diaphragm.

8 a Brodie's abscess.
  b Indolent localised staphylococcal bone infection.

9, 700 and 701
  a Syphilis. He has now developed secondary syphilis.
  b Mucous patches (these may coalesce, giving rise to 'snail track'
    ulcers).
  c Yes.

02 and 703
  a Osteochondritis of
    i) the lunate (Keinboch's disease)
    ii) the navicular (Kohler's disease).
  b Both conditions are thought to arise as a result of aseptic necrosis of
    the ossification centre with subsequent reparation.
  c No. Complete recovery is usual.

704 a A keloid.

     b Negroes (especially female) have a higher risk than Caucasians. Oth
       risk groups include patient's with Turner's and Noonan's syndromes
       and acromegaly. A family history may sometimes be elicited.

705 a Central ulcerative keratitis with abscess formation.

     b Streptococcus pneumoniae, Staphylococcus aureus and Pseudomon
       aeruginosa.

706 and 707

     a Charcot joints.

     b i)   Syringomyelia.
       ii) Diabetes mellitus.
       iii) Neurosyphilis.

     c Scars from old (painless) cuts and burns

708 a Muscle wasting of upper thighs.

     b Diabetic amyotrophy.

     c No specific treatment other than control of glycaemia by convention
       means.

709 a Palmar erythema.

     b Thyrotoxicosis.

     c i)   Pretibial myxoedema.
       ii) Cutaneous vasodilatation and excessive sweating.
       iii) Melanin pigmentation (increased adenocorticotrophic hormone
           production).
       iv) Alopecia.
       v) Onycholysis.

710 and 711

     a Syndesmophyte formation.

     b Psoriatic spondyloarthropathy.

     c Natal cleft, umbilicus, genitalia.

712 a Bronchography.

     b Extensive saccular bronchiectasis (with saccule formation in proxima
       bronchi).

     c Aspergillus.

     d i)   Early (type I) reaction after prick test with aspergillus fumigatus
           extract.
       ii) Late (type III, Arthus) reaction after four to ten hours.

713 a i)   Atrophic glossitis.
       ii) Angular stomatitis.

     b Malabsorption of iron may be solely responsible but there may also b
       vitamin B_{12} deficiency.

     c A blood film. The normal mean corpuscular volume may mask a
       dimorphic red cell picture and the polymorphs may show nuclear
       hypersegmentation.

14 and 716
    a i) 'Corkscrew' hairs.
       ii) Patchy discolouration.
    b Vitamin C deficiency.

15 a S1, S2, S3 syndrome.
    b It may occur normally when it reflects the juvenile pattern of right
       ventricular predominance; or in right ventricular hypertrophy.

17 a It has a left lower motor neurone facial palsy.
    b Forceps delivery.
    c If traumatic, full recovery is the rule. Failure of recovery usually
       indicates an atraumatic aetiology such as agenesis of the facial
       nucleus.

18 a Widened intercondylar notch.
    b Haemophilia.

19 a Arteriovenous fistula.
       (Proximal venous obstruction less likely in the absence of oedema).
    b i) Surgical (eg for haemodialysis).
       ii) Traumatic (accidental, self-inflicted).

20 a Peutz-Jegher syndrome.
    b i) Intestinal obstruction.
       ii) Intestinal haemorrhage.

21 and 722
    a i) Loss of joint space.
       ii) Periarticular sclerosis.
       iii) Subarticular cyst formation.
       iv) Marginal osteophytes.
    b i) Pain, especially on weight bearing (unless these are 'neuropathic'
         joints).
       ii) Stiffness after periods of rest ('gelling').

23 a Herald patch.
    b Pityriasis rosea.

24 a Vasculitis.
    b i) Perforated peptic ulcer (or other bowel perforation), secondary to
         non-steroidal anti-inflammatory or steroid drug therapy.
       ii) Intestinal infarction.
       iii) Gall bladder infarction.
       iv) Pancreatic infarction.

725 a Right IIIrd nerve palsy.

b In the right paramedian mid-brain involving the red nucleus and the nucleus of the IIIrd nerve.

c Claude's syndrome (Benedikt's syndrome if there is also contralateral sensory impairment).

726 a Gas in the biliary tree; distal small bowel distension.

b Gallstone ileus.

c No. The gallstone is usually a large radiolucent cholesterol stone.

727 a 1 Tooth in a dermoid cyst.

2 Fat/fluid level within the cyst.

3 Iliac crest.

4 Right psoas muscle.

b Fat.

728 a Yes; oral ulceration is typically found after paraquat ingestion.

b i) Gastric lavage with instillation of Fuller's earth.

ii) Assay of blood and urine for paraquat to confirm the diagnosis and assess the severity of poisoning.

iii) Measurement of baseline renal function, hepatic and lung function.

iv) Charcoal haemoperfusion ($\pm$ prostacyclin to minimise platelet loss) or haemodialysis may be employed to enhance clearance of paraquat but have not been shown to reduce mortality in man.

v) Avoidance of oxygen supplementation.

c Radiotherapy was dramatically successful in a single patient who developed widespread fibrosis. This therapy remains to be verified by a proper clinical trial.

729 a Continuous murmur(s) over the chest.

b Pulmonary arteriovenous anomaly associated with hereditary haemorrhagic telangiectasia (Rendu-Osler-Weber syndrome).

730 a i) Cardiomegaly.

ii) Upper lobe pulmonary venous distension.

iii) Basal Kerley 'B' lines.

iv) Hilar haze of alveolar oedema.

b Loop diuretic.

731 a Scabies.

b By identification of burrows (particularly wrists, interdigital clefts) and demonstration of scabies mite.

c i) After bathing, application of a scabiecide (eg. benzyl benzoate, gamma benzene hexachloride).

ii) Treatment of family contacts.

32 a Central retinal venous thrombosis.
   b i)   Retinal arteriosclerotic nipping (the commonest cause) — may
           be underlying hypertension, hyperlipidaemia, diabetes mellitus.
     ii) Retinal phlebitis.
     iii) Hyperviscosity syndrome (eg. macroglobulinaemia,
           polycythaemia).
     iv) Glaucoma.
   c Secondary glaucoma.

33 and 734
   a i)   Bilateral exophthalmos, asymmetrical proptosis (right eye more
           than left), conjunctival swelling and suffusion.
     ii) Nodular lesions and oedema, consistent with infiltrative
           dermopathy (pretibial myxoedema).
   b Graves' (Basedow's) disease.
   c i)   diffuse goitre
     ii) thyrotoxicosis.

35 a Failure of the mandibular arch to develop normally during
       embryogenesis.
   b Treacher-Collins syndrome (craniofacial dysostosis).
   c The malleus and incus. The stapes develops from the second branchial
       arch.

36 a Calcification of the supraspinatus tendon.
   b An arc of painful movement on active shoulder abduction.
   c Passive movements are usually normal.

37 and 738
   a i)   Target lesions typical of erythema multiforme.
     ii) Diffuse nodular pulmonary opacities suggestive of viral,
           chlamydial, or mycoplasma pneumonia.
   b The underlying infection may be solely responsible. Antibiotic
       therapy may result in drug allergy eg sulphonamides, penicillins,
       tetracyclines. The radiological changes may be secondary to erythema
       multiforme alone.

39 a They lie between the periostium (pericranium) and skull and are
       bounded by the sutures.
   b A cephalhaematoma never crosses the mid line, unlike a caput
       succedaneum.
   c No. Spontaneous resorption without residual deformity will occur.

40 a Black hairy tongue; there is overgrowth of the filiform papillae and
       the discolouration is due to tobacco, chromogenic bacteria or
       Aspergillus niger.
   b Oral antibiotics; smoking or chewing tobacco.
   c Amphotericin B may be helpful in Aspergillus infection.

41 a Mongolian blue spot.
   b No abnormality, since there is no association with spina bifida.

742 a Pathological cupping of the optic disc. (The disc is also pale).
 b Chronic simple glaucoma.
 c Tonometry.
 d Exaggeration of the normal diurnal variation in intra ocular pressure (a single measurement may well be normal. Eventually the pressure will become persistently raised).

743 a Nodular panniculitis.
 b Pancreas.

744 Venous gangrene, secondary to deep venous thrombosis.

745 a Acne rosacea.
 b i) Acne vulgaris.
   ii) Seborrhoeic dermatitis.
   iii) Perioral dermatitis.
   iv) Systemic lupus erythematosus.

746 a Flea bites.
 b Microscope examination of brushings from skin, clothes (inner surfaces, seams), household pets, house dust for pulex irritans, the human flea.

747 a Wenckebach phenomenon.
 b Recent inferior myocardial infarction (ST elevation in leads II and III).
 c No. It may be seen in association with high vagal tone such as athlete

748 a i) Thyrotoxic myopathy.
   ii) Carcinomatous myopathy.
   iii) Others — polymyositis, progressive muscular atrophy.
 b Exophthalmos and lid retraction are suggestive of thyrotoxicosis.
 c Serum thyroxine and tri-iodothyronine measurement.
 d Radioactive iodine therapy or antithyroid drugs. (Surgery not appropriate in absence of large goitre).

749 a Haemorrhages, exudates in a segmental distribution.
 b Superior temporal branch retinal venous occlusion.
 c Poor. (Venous return from the macula is generally interrupted).

750 a Causes of symmetrical macroglossia include —
   i) Acromegaly.
   ii) Hypothyroidism.
   iii) Primary amyloidosis.
   iv) Down's syndrome.

751 a Haemorrhagic chickenpox.
 b Defect in cell-mediated immunity.
 c By demonstration of cutaneous anergy (eg. lack of response to Mantoux test).

52 a Eczema craquele (asteatotic eczema).
   b Underlying malignancy particularly·lymphoma of the gastrointestinal tract; hypothyroidism; zinc deficiency; essential fatty acid deficiency. A more localised form occurs on the shins particularly in elderly patients in winter.

53 a Angiokeratoma. These are not lesions of Kaposi's sarcoma.
   b None.

54 a A — Large right pleural effusion.
      B — Posterior aspect of right lung.
   b Ovarian fibroma (ovarian carcinoma less likely).

55 a Sturge-Weber syndrome.
   b i) Meninges.
      ii) Eye.
   c Intracranial calcification.

56 a Right middle lobe consolidation.
   b Assuming patent right middle lobe bronchus.
      i)   Bronchial breath sounds.
      ii) Bronchophony.
      iii) Whispering pectoriloquy.

57 a Early development of secondary sex characteristics, pubic hair.
   b Precocious puberty.
   c Darkening and rugosity of the scrotal skin.

58 a Multiple retinal scars from photocoagulation therapy for diabetic retinopathy.
   b i) Clofibrate (for hard exudates).
      ii) Pituitary ablation.
          (Diabetic control, if poor, should be improved).

59 a Molluscum contagiosum.
   b These include expression, curettage, cryotherapy, podophyllin/ ethanol paint.

60 a Close her eyes and mouth tightly shut.
   b Bell's phenomenon.
   c Stylomastoid foramen.

1 and 762
   a $IIIB_s$.
   b Combination chemotherapy such as MVPP (mustine, vinblastine, procarbazine and prednisolone).
   c Reed-Sternberg giant cells with characteristic "mirror-image" nuclei are considered to be necessary to make the diagnosis.

763 Neither. This appearance, of gangrene with demarcation, does not develop until several days after the original injury. Treatment at this stage is conservative and consists in keeping the affected areas dry and free of infection.

764 a Intracerebral haemorrhage in the right cerebral hemisphere.
   b No. Her hypertension is most probably a consequence of the intracerebral haemorrhage and immediate hypotensive therapy may considerably impair cerebral perfusion.

765 a Stomatocytosis.
   b Alcoholic liver disease; high-dose phenothiazine (especially chlorpromazine) administration; familial inheritance.
   c Impaired transport of sodium through the cell membrane.

766 a i) Subcutaneous emphysema.
      ii) Mediastinal emphysema (aortic arch).
      iii) Intubated left pneumothorax.
   b This varies with respiration — from approximately -10 cm H_2O to -4 cm H_2O during quiet inspiration and expiration.

767 a Goitre.
   b Hypothyroidism.
   c Autoimmune thyroiditis (Hashimoto's disease). Other causes include iodine deficiency and drug-induced goitrous hypothyroidism (eg lithium or para-aminosalicylic acid).

768 a Necrotising nodular scleritis (the nodules have the typical histological appearance of rheumatoid nodules).
   b Scleral necrosis, with exposure of the uvea (similar to scleromalacia perforans, which is typically a painless necrosis).

769 a Alopecia areata.
      (Nail pitting and thickening are commonly seen in association with this disorder).
   b Approximately 1 in 2.

770 a Digital infarcts due to vasculitis.
   b Connective tissue disease, particularly systemic lupus erythematosus or scleroderma; cryoglobulinaemia; polyarteritis nodosa; infective endocarditis; hypersensitivity to drugs.

771 and 772
   a Osteopetrosis (Albers-Schönberg disease, Marble Bone disease).
   b Autosomal recessive (a milder, autosomal dominant form exists).
   c The mandible (as can be seen on the skull x-ray).
   d Bone marrow transplantation.

773 a Yaws due to treponema pertenue.
   b None.

774 a Syphilis — primary chancre.
    b Dark field examination of fluid expressed from the ulcer
    c The Fluorescent Treponemal Antibody Test.

775 and 776
      i)   Chickenpox.
      ii)   Oral candidiasis.

INDEX